Healing Through Worship

Some other books by Dr. Hutchison:

THE CHURCH AND
SPIRITUAL HEALING   Rider & Co., 1955 (out of print)

A FAITH TO LIVE BY   W. A. Wilde, USA, 1959 (out of print)

SCOTTISH PUBLIC
EDUCATIONAL DOCUMENTS   S.C.R.E., 1973

KIRK LIFE IN OLD CARMUNNOCK   Carmunnock Kirk Session, 1978

GOD BELIEVES IN YOU!   Eyre & Spottiswoode, 1980

CARMUNNOCK
CHURCH, 1854 – 1948   Carmunnock Kirk Session, 1980

WELL, I'M BLESSED!   Eyre & Spottiswoode, 1981

HAVE A WORD WITH GOD   Eyre & Spottiswoode, 1981

Healing Through Worship

by

HARRY HUTCHISON

First published in 1981 by
Eyre & Spottiswoode (Publishers) Ltd.
North Way, Andover, Hampshire SP10 5BE
© 1980 Harry Hutchison
ISBN 0 413 80190 X
Printed by T. J. Press (Padstow) Ltd.
Padstow, Cornwall

CONTENTS

Dr. Henry Hutchison was born in Alloa, Clackmannanshire, and attended Dollar Academy where he was Athletics Champion as well as Dux Medallist. For a few years he played cricket for Clackmannan County. After a period of War Service in the Royal Air Force, he completed his M.A. and B.D. Degrees at Edinburgh University, and later gained the B.Ed. of Toronto University and the M.Litt. and Ph.D. Degrees of Glasgow University. He is a trained teacher and holds Diplomas in Music and in Religious Education.

His first charge as a Minister of the Church of Scotland was in Saltcoats, Ayrshire. He moved to Glasgow for a few years before accepting a Call to St. Paul's Presbyterian Church, Peterborough, Ontario—one of the largest Presbyterian congregations in Canada. On returning to Scotland he became involved in the teaching of religion in schools, but in 1967 he was appointed Lecturer in Education at Glasgow University.

Eventually deciding to move back into parish work, he was inducted to the historic parish of Carmunnock in 1977. He has contributed to many Journals—several of his articles and sermons, for example, having appeared in the *Expository Times* and in *The Christian Ministry* (USA)—and the titles of some of his books are noted elsewhere in the present volume. He is married, with one son who holds a Major Open Scholarship at Oxford.

FOREWORD

In a Foreword which Dr. Geoffrey Evans wrote for
Dr. Leslie Weatherhead's well-known book on
Psychology, Religion, and Healing, published
nearly thirty years ago, he made the simple
statement that "the majority of doctors, and
certainly psychologists, would agree with the
author that much of our physical health depends
on our spiritual health". There are still some
today who would dispute this, but to the vast
majority the truth of the statement is self-evident.
Certainly for the present little volume this is the
indispensable basis of all that will be said. As the
American novelist Nathaniel Hawthorne once
wrote: "A bodily disease, which we look upon as
whole and entire within itself, may, after all, be
but a symptom of some ailment in the spiritual
part".

In Part I of the book we begin by taking a brief
look at the context of non-physical healing and
highlighting the challenge which is thrown out by
the undeniable fact that people are healed
through worship today; and since there seem to be
so many misguided notions as to the place of
sickness in people's lives (notions held by some
Christians as well as non-Christians!), some

i

attempt is made in chapter 2 to present what the author believes to be a balanced and positive view. The basic claim, of course, is that God wills health for all His people, and that to fight sickness is to engage in a Christlike work.

> "Empower the hands and hearts and wills
> Of friends in lands afar,
> Who battle with the body's ills,
> And wage *Thy* holy war."

But it's not just in lands afar, but in this land too, that the holy war must be fought. And it's here and everywhere that we must stress the fact that, as Jesus Himself made clear in the Gospel, the ultimate purpose of any healings that take place is to "glorify God". A bodily healing that doesn't lead to increased spiritual wellbeing is incomplete.

Part I concludes with a short discussion of various aspects of personal religion in so far as they seem to be important for any possibility of healing through worship, and Part II consists of the 25 Healing Services themselves, prefaced by a brief explanation of how they are intended to be used in private devotion. May those who use them not only know that

> "Thine arm, O Lord, in days of old,
> Was strong to heal and save",

but also that He is "our great Deliverer still"!

H.H.

The Manse of Carmunnock,
August, 1981

PART I

Chapter 1

THE CONTEXT AND THE CHALLENGE

In his book *The Liberal Imagination,* Lionel Trilling rather bluntly but strikingly commented: "We are all ill: but even a universal sickness implies an idea of health". It's this positive idea of health which must be the context within which Christians can best consider the whole question of healing through worship—or, indeed, any method of healing.

It goes without saying, of course, that healing through orthodox medical treatment will, in the foreseeable future, continue to be the most common form of healing in our society. (Wasn't it Seneca, in the first century, who commented: "It is medicine, not scenery, for which a sick man must go on searching"?) And the Christian certainly will continue to be grateful for the enormous medical benefits open to him today. But there is little doubt in the present writer's mind that the Church's potentially powerful ministry of healing is seriously undervalued and under-used — and this includes healing through one's own private devotions.

Despite the flood of publications on "faith healing" during the past few decades — or perhaps because of the excesses and extravagant claims to be found in some of them — large numbers of professing Christians continue to disregard the very powerful challenge which a serious reading of the New Testament might highlight. The Synoptic Gospels all stress that Christ's commission to his disciples was concerned not only with teaching and preaching, but with healing too. As Alan Richardson has noted in *The Miracle Stories of the Gospels*, we have plenty of "first-hand evidence that, from the earliest days, the ministry of healing was placed side by side with that of preaching in the missionary labours of the Church".

Now it's true, of course, that some denominations of the Church have placed more emphasis on a healing ministry than others, and that some prominent individual healers have come to the fore during the last decade or two to exercise what some people might regard as a spectacular healing ministry. This side of things has had generous coverage both in newspaper articles and in the case-history type of book. But considerably less has so far been said about healing through private devotions — and it's this aspect of healing which will concern us mainly in the present volume. It is to the individual worshipper who seeks healing through prayer, just as much as to the "famous" healer, that Christ's words apply. "Truly, I say to you, he who believes in me will also do the works that I do; and greater works than these will he do, because I go to the Father" (Jn.14.12). Healing through worship is a possibility simply because it's Christ the Healer with whom the worshipper is in contact.

No doubt one comes across the fairly common assertion that, whatever place might be found for a ministry of healing within the context of the modern Church, the actual "results" could never be as spectacular as those healings recorded, for example, in the Book of Acts. This is a view that is worth trying to resist. No doubt the Christian may hold this view out of a misplaced reverence for the period of Christian history covered by the Acts. He ascribes a sanctity to this period which he won't allow to the modern one. Perhaps he even feels that, if spectacular healings took place in the present age, something of the uniqueness and authority of the New Testament might be lost for him. What an unfortunate viewpoint! Christ repeats: "He who believes in me will also do the works that I do; and greater works than these will he do, because I go to the Father".

Sometimes it's difficult not to have a slight suspicion that the modern Church's refusal — and the individual Christian's refusal — to face the challenge of the Early Church's healing ministry is grounded in her self-satisfaction, or even her complacency, at putting all, or almost all, the stress on a "spiritual" gospel. Such people would claim that physical healing was of little importance beside the salvation of the soul. It is one of the beliefs of the present writer that a proper attitude towards healing through worship can lead to the ultimate blessing of spiritual wholeness—but this is certainly not to dismiss physical healing as a matter of little or no importance. Physical health "is the second blessing that we mortals are capable of", wrote Izaak Walton. But let no man suggest that it isn't a blessing devoutly to be wished!

By all means let us seek this blessing wherever it may be found—be it through medical science or any other channel. But, as L. W. Grensted wrote a few decades ago in his *Psychology and God*, "while the Church is waiting for more knowledge, taking counsel with doctors and psychologists, seeking to understand the kinds of disorder which may be expected to yield to spiritual treatment, it may well be that she should rather be praying, 'Lord, increase our faith'." Without this context of faith the Church may well continue to be ineffective in her healing ministry, and individual Christians who suffer from ill-health may well be unable to find the urge and the confidence to seek healing through worship.

The Bible suggests that "the Kingdom of God is within you". If people could appreciate that fact better, perhaps their marvelling when healing "miracles" do occur would change to a humble but joyful acceptance of an order of things that was meant to be far more normal than most people realise. To accept the Gospel which brings us into fellowship with God is, at the same time, to accept the promise of healing which, in some substantial form, the same God offers through that fellowship. It is not without significance that the *British Medical Journal*, some years ago, stated categorically that "no tissue of the human body is wholly removed from the influence of spirit". That's a statement which is both a challenge to, and an invitation to, faith!

That point is stressed too by Leslie Weatherhead in his book *Psychology, Religion, and Healing*. "The human being is a very closely-knit unity of body, mind, and spirit. In such a unity there cannot be disease at any point, at any level of being, without the whole personality being to some extent affected." No doubt some of us know the effect of indigestion on our tempers! But it's not every Christian who is prepared to acknowledge that spiritual disharmony may cause mental and physical disharmony, and that the healing of mental or physical ailments may not be possible without the healing of the spirit.

Many sufferers who seek healing through

worship could do worse than ask themselves: "What spiritual disharmony may have led to my physical illness?" The answer may be "None"; but simply to be aware of this unity of body, mind, and spirit can, as a general rule, be a valuable step forward in one's quest for healing through private devotions. Certainly "health" isn't merely a state of physical wellbeing; nor is "salvation" something which concerns the soul only. No doubt Emerson was unduly simplifying when he suggested: "The best part of health is fine disposition", but assuredly one's "disposition" vis-à-vis God is an absolutely crucial factor in one's total sense of wellbeing. In fact, the closer one is to God, the more likely one is to experience that wholeness which God Himself desires for all His people.

Chapter 2

SOME WRONG IDEAS ABOUT SICKNESS

To get close to God may be rather difficult if we are mistaken as to His true nature. And any possibilities of healing through worship will be grasped fully only when we have clarified our minds about this divine nature. Certainly to have a wrong idea about God's will, as far as sickness is concerned, must have a substantial effect on the "usefulness" of seeking healing through private devotions.

It's surely one of the curious tricks of human thought that people should be able sincerely to believe in the presence of illness as part of the positive and deliberate will of God. What irony that the very Scriptures which first told the world of a God of Love also create a "problem" for the Christian. To the non-Christian, of course, to the man who doesn't believe in the God of Love, sickness or evil isn't a problem at all. He may believe either that illness is the result of a god's malice or that no god had anything to do with

7

it — and he's content to leave it at that. But not the Christian. For him there's a real problem.

By and large, this "problem" was much less acute for the people of the Old Testament. The early Jews — and particularly during the period between the Old and New Testaments — tended to believe, however hesitantly, that sickness was often God's will for man; and although some attention was paid in early Israel to the alleviation of sickness, it was rather slight. True, the Rabbis did sometimes pray for a patient's recovery. True, material remedies for illness were sometimes used. But the dominant belief was that sickness came because God willed it. Most Jews certainly saw health as an indication of divine favour, and sickness as an equally clear indication of divine disfavour. Indeed, many people regarded material remedies as little else than an impious interference with the purposes of God.

Is it possible that some Christians find a sanction for their idea of sickness as God's will in this Jewish belief? If so, it's strange that they don't consider the evidence of the New Testament and of the practices of the Early Church. That Church certainly gave little encouragement either to the belief that material remedies should be avoided, or to the general view of sickness as God's will. Her ministry of healing provides the strongest evidence of the fact that she repudiated the views that were common at that time among the Jews and among other peoples. One wonders whether the relative absence of a healing ministry in the Church today is due, in part, to the sneaking feeling that sickness may well be God's will for some people.

If we glance at Christ's own practice of healing, it's perfectly clear that He saw no contradiction in using both material remedies and non-material ones. And He surely exploded the whole idea that God ordains sickness for anybody. Whatever elements in the universe may be responsible for creating disease, whether they are spiritual or physical in origin, they are to be ruthlessly eliminated by those whose desire is to do the will of God. Christ saw God's ideal purpose for man as health of body, mind, and spirit; and the fact that such health was rarely attained didn't in any way affect His working for it and believing in it.

To the early Jewish view that the healing of the sick was usually "against nature", Jesus set His own view that it's *sickness* which is abnormal, not health. Sixty years ago the Lambeth Report on the Healing Ministry of the Christian Church contained a splendid statement of the belief which must lie behind our approach to the whole subject of healing through worship. "Health is God's primary will for all His children, and disease is not only to be combated, but to be combated in God's name as a way of carrying out His will. However disease may be brought about, and in whatever way it may be overruled for good, it is in itself an evil."

One simple story in the New Testament— Luke, chapter 13, verses 10 to 17—is enough to show that Christ refused to accept illness as part of the kingdom of evil. Rather did He regard it as His specific mission to subjugate that kingdom. This story in itself is a powerful answer to those who believe their illness to be "divinely sent". Christ didn't deny the *problem* of evil; but He did deny the *necessity* of evil. If, then, a sufferer is unwilling to surrender his belief that sickness is God's will for him, healing through worship must be a very long shot indeed! As the present writer said over twenty-five years ago in his *The Church and Spiritual Healing,* we must "share the conviction that healing is always unimpeded from the divine side, from the side of Nature. That which prevents it from penetrating into body, mind, or spirit, is on the human side." This isn't to suggest that man is to blame, but simply to assert the vital principle that God doesn't ordain sickness for anyone.

There's another principle worth stating, if healing through worship is to have its full potential. Sickness mustn't be regarded as a direct punishment for sin; though this, of course, was another commonly held view in Old

Testament times. To most Jews at that time sickness wasn't simply an arbitrary evidence of God's disfavour, but a deserved punishment for sin! Health, likewise, was regarded not simply as a sign of God's favour, but also as a reward for righteousness. Is it surprising in this context to find that the Jews weren't distinguished as medical men? Their medical backwardness was certainly due, in large part, to this prevalent notion of illness being the direct result of some family or personal sin.

Now this isn't to minimise the progress that they had, in fact, made in the medical sphere. The Talmud mentions, among other things, a regular treatment for wounds (wine, oil, and bandaging), a form of what is now called Caesarean section, and amputations. And, of course, when we compare Israel with her neighbouring nations, we must be impressed with the careful hygienic precautions of the Mosaic period. But their medical advances would surely have been even more impressive had they not held on to their basic belief in sickness as, in some sense, a punishment from God. This "heresy", as we may rightly call it, is illustrated in the well-known query which some Jews addressed to Jesus. "Rabbi, who sinned, this man or his parents, that he should be born blind?" The questioners took it for granted that the man's blindness would be due to some specific sin, committed either by his parents or by himself.

Christ's reply is significant. "Neither this man nor his parents sinned" (John 9.3. N.I.V.). No doubt this would come as something of a shock to His hearers—and it probably had a considerable therapeutic influence on the blind man himself. Jesus flatly denied, in *this* case, that suffering was directly related to sin. And when, on occasion, He spoke of illness as the work of "Satan", whether or not He was merely using the terminology of the time, He would in fact be making it even clearer to the Jews that illness was not deserved, since an indwelling of Satan was, to most Jews, purely fortuitous and reflected in no way upon the "possessed" person. When Jesus asked: "Shouldn't this woman whom Satan has bound be loosed from this bond?", His hearers would certainly be reluctant to give up their belief that her illness was a punishment for sin—and one can imagine how angry they would be to have their cherished but misguided beliefs repudiated.

Christians today are surely invited not to be among those who, as Leslie Weatherhead once put it, "still cling to the heresy that illness is handed out to people by an offended God". They mustn't be of those who subscribe to "the old bogey that suffering is God's chastisement and that the sufferer must bow beneath the rod". This, of course, isn't to deny that some sickness may well be *self*-inflicted (many drunkards, for example, bring upon themselves various serious illnesses), but this is something quite different from the idea that God inflicts a person with some illness or other. God doesn't punish us; we punish ourselves. As Rebecca Beard noted in her *Everyman's Search*: "Physical science has changed our thinking. We cannot think of God punishing us any more than we can conceive of electricity deliberately punishing anyone. Our ignorance of the law will not save us if we touch the exposed end of a live wire. We put *ourselves* out of the Garden of Eden."

There's just one further wrong idea about sickness that must concern us briefly in this chapter. Some people apparently believe in the necessity of illness as part of God's disciplining of man; and yet, oddly enough, such people usually do not fail to summon a doctor with all speed when sickness does come! And surely their doing so is an instinctive repudiation of the idea of sickness as God's chosen vehicle of the "perfecting of His saints". Despite the New Testament idea that the "Old Adam" is to be mortified so that the soul may be more fully alive, the general evidence of the Bible points clearly to the fact that the redemption of the body is a legitimate and desirable aim.

No doubt some people may claim that Christ's own perfecting through suffering is a confirmation of the idea that God ordains sickness to "perfect" men and women. But such a claim would be unjustified. Christ's suffering was not that of sickness or disease. There is no mention in the Gospel that Christ was ever ill. His suffering was rather the inevitable result of His unique spirituality. He suffered because He felt so deeply for mankind. In no sense can the Cross be called a sickness sent by God.

Moreover, the picture of Christ in the Gospel is in strong contrast to the morbid asceticism which has manifested itself at different periods of the Church's history. True religious discipline is attained neither through God-sent disease nor through self-inflicted pain. It's with all reverence that we might suggest that many of the Church's saints have suffered so much because of their conviction that suffering was necessary to their perfecting. We don't deny, of course, that God *can* use sickness and suffering of all kinds for His own glory and for man's blessedness. We don't deny that people, by a right attitude to illness, can become "saints". But it remains true that, if sickness were an indispensable condition of Christian saintliness and perfection, Christ would have refrained from fighting it. In any case, the presence of sickness has never, in itself, moulded people into saints. It's their reaction to it that has done so. A person may certainly find, after an experience of illness, that he has developed a nobler character than he had before the illness took place. But the question still remains: "How much more noble *might* it have been if expressed in a completely healthy and harmonised body?"

For all the errors and inconsistencies of Christian Science, there is one considerable service rendered by it, namely, its strenuous opposition to the idea that saintliness is inevitably bound up with sickness. There is, in fact, nothing in illness itself which guarantees Christian fortitude and saintliness. Dr. Weatherhead, in his *Psychology, Religion, and Healing*, has written one of the most succinct and powerful statements on this theme. "It is thought by some that suffering makes saints. It is more likely to make rebellious cynics or querulous neurotics. The saints have not been made saints because of suffering, but in spite of it. It has been their reaction to suffering that made saintliness, not the suffering itself. No word must be said to belittle the great saintliness of some characters, but if they could have been as fully awakened spiritually without physical disability, then, as instruments in the hand of God, they would have been of even greater usefulness through health than through disease. The matter can be put briefly: Jesus would not have been more holy if He had been the victim of disease. God does not *need* evil before He can accomplish His maximum good."

Now, of course, some sick people have done more for the world than others who enjoyed the best of physical health. And certainly a physically sick man need not have a sick soul. But that doesn't contradict Christ's own belief that a man who was whole in body, mind, and spirit was potentially the most effective power for good, as well as the embodiment of God's own will for mankind.

Perhaps it's worth remembering also that a man's religion may actually be keeping him ill! Many a neurotic suffers illness with morbid satisfaction — so many medical practitioners and psychologists tell us — and in that situation the idea of being "perfected through suffering" is a most convenient rationalisation! So often it's because a person doesn't want to be cured that he thereby automatically blocks the healing energies of God. And, by a vicious circle, his distorted view of God becomes even more distorted.

However, all that has been said here in no way contradicts the idea that the "secondary" will of God is that a sick man should so react to illness as to win spiritual triumph from it. In this sense, sickness *may* be a discipline. But it is still of the greatest importance to insist that God's "primary" will is the fullest health. Only such a view gives due honour to God. Only such a view gives people their maximum chance of recovery. As has been said: "It's not wicked to be ill, but it's wicked to be more ill than you need be".

Chapter 3

THE REAL PURPOSE OF HEALING
THROUGH WORSHIP

It is worth saying at the beginning of this chapter that no claim is being made that all sicknesses should be able to be cured through worship. In many cases medical treatment is — or would seem to be — the most obvious and most "sensible" one to seek. A man riddled with bullets would be somewhat more likely to respond to an operation than to prayers said for him — though the latter would certainly be far from superfluous. It's not just the businessmen who, as Norman Vincent Peale notes, "are discovering that one of the greatest efficiency methods is prayer power". But, when that is acknowledged, we must also admit that perhaps even the closest fellowship between a man and his God may not be able to cure everything. We simply don't at the moment know how limitless the possibilities are — though they are almost certainly greater than we imagine. As Tennyson commented: "More things are wrought by prayer than this world dreams of".

But the point we want to highlight in this chapter is the one that concerns the ultimate purpose behind healing through prayer—or, indeed, behind *any* form of healing. And St. Luke's story of the Ten Lepers may give us considerable insight into this question (ch.17). The story tells us that they were all healed, and so why condemn the nine "thankless ones"? What point was there in Jesus saying: "Your faith has made you whole"? The clue to the story undoubtedly lies in the meaning of the word "whole". Jesus was, of course, interested in the bodily healing, but was He not even more interested in the personal wholeness? The *Interpreter's Bible* certainly takes this view. "Perhaps the word 'whole' means whole of more than the leprosy. We must doubt if the nine lepers were any better *men* because of their cure. Were they not worse off through their ingratitude? The ingratitude was a worse leprosy than the physical disease. But the Samaritan, because of his praising God, was really whole, in soul as well as in body, for eternity as well as for time."

It's difficult not to endorse this conclusion. Christ's overriding aim was always to bring spiritual health, which, in turn, would be a major factor in securing or maintaining physical health. As the *Dictionary of Christ and the Gospels* puts it: "The action of Jesus was upon the complex personality, body and spirit, but upon the body through the spirit. His power went directly to the central life, to the man, to the living person, and this may be traced in all His dealings with disease and infirmity, both of body and of mind." Christ's purpose was to nourish faith in *Himself*, not to cause a mere sense of relief in the healed person. The purpose of Christ's healings, indeed, is no different from the purpose of all other parts of the Gospel tradition, i.e. to evoke or deepen man's under-standing of the true Person of Christ. The healing "miracles" were not just *tours de force*; and certainly Jesus was not a little distressed when a demonstration of power through heal-ing failed to evoke the response of faith in the healed person. Indeed, as St. John suggests (6.26), Jesus felt that, without the response of "glorifying God", the healing miracles were profitless, and their purpose utterly frustrated. The temptation is ever with us of using our religion as a solution of our temporal problems, and caring far more for that than for the glory of God. Those who seek healing through worship might be wise to ponder on that fact!

In his *Miracle Stories of the Gospels*, Alan Richardson insists that, "apart from this faith in Jesus, the miracles of Jesus, even though our intellects were convinced on scientific grounds that they had taken place, could have no more meaning for us than they had for those in the multitude who stood by and were amazed". The most important thing in healing through prayer (or through any other agency) is the spiritual change, the new belief in the power of God, the new conviction of the love of God. Without evoking that, the real purpose of the healing is unfulfilled — though, of course, this isn't to say that we cannot be glad of any partial healing that has taken place. But the Church must never simply promise physical healing. We must never promise that such healing will take place through personal devotions. The aim — and the hope — is that the whole man will be brought to God. We are invited to believe not in a wonder-worker but a Saviour.

Christ's own unwillingness to give "signs" as evidence of his divinity is mentioned time and again in the New Testament. And it's equally obvious that, for the writers of that book, the significance of the healings lay not in their "wonder-content" but in their spiritual reference. Every healing was a pointer to the fact that the power of God was being made available as never before. Healings are stressed in the New Testament not because they are wonderful works, but because of the Church's conviction that, in this one Man of Nazareth, the unique powers of a New Age were seen and heard. The Church believed then, and must believe now, that the power to save the body and the power to save the soul was the same power. The preached word and the healing works were evidences of a redemption which went far beyond the conception of redemption shared by Christ's contemporaries — and indeed far beyond the conception of redemption shared by the Church of today.

Chapter 4

HEALING AND PERSONAL RELIGION (i)

As we've already tried to make clear, the idea of healing through worship as a kind of short cut to health is a travesty of its whole purpose. Such healing normally rests on a conscientious spiritual discipline on the part of the person seeking healing, but this is not, of course, the same as saying that everything depends on the patient. Some "faith healers" unfortunately give this impression; but there are very few people who have the spiritual resources to "heal themselves"! The general principle that the most effective healing comes where man has contributed something to it must not be allowed to degenerate into the unwarranted idea that he should contribute everything.

Clearly, then, we must state our conviction that healing through worship is not a method which demands less cooperation from the patient than medical healing. It demands considerably more. We don't deny, of course, that God can "save" a man suddenly, any more than we would deny He can heal suddenly; but God's normal healing method does seem to be a process rather than a sudden act. As Christopher Woodard wrote many years ago: "I feel that the 'making whole' comes not by sudden spasmodic outpouring of the healing spirit, but by a continuous flow of it" *(A Doctor Heals by Faith)*. For people who want quick results, this isn't a popular idea! But perhaps God is more interested in thoroughness than in speed.

It's certainly true that, in sickness, a whole process of growth, involving the breaking down of the illness and the building up of tissue, may be necessary for complete healing; and it would surely be unreasonable for us to *expect* this process to be compressed into one spectacular moment of healing—even though this does seem to happen on occasion. Moreover, one wonders whether instantaneous healings carry the "danger" that they may deprive the patient of a gradual building up of his prayer life. Spiritual discipline and true healing are intimately connected in the vast majority of cases.

Perhaps it goes without saying that this spiritual discipline must be geared to a personal faith in Christ. The faith which is required of a patient interested in healing through worship is not simply faith to be healed, but faith in the

Person of Jesus Christ. After all, how can one suddenly manufacture a faith that he is going to be healed? Such a belief must surely be the product of a relationship already established, and one in which the element of personal trust is primary. The faith which we are called on to have, in fact, is the faith which is essential not just in face of bodily sickness, but in face of *all* life's situations.

It is, of course, true that the New Testament mentions several occasions on which Jesus seemed prepared to grant a healing to people who had only a very superficial faith. But Jesus knew better than anyone that, in these cases, a "cure" in the sense of the healing of body, mind, and spirit had not been achieved. Christ never refused the measure of healing which was possible in face of a man's condition; but, in the long run, He couldn't contradict His own law that bodily and mental healing depend, in an intimate way, on the state of the soul. Anything less than a "saving" faith meant *something* less than a complete healing.

The story of Blind Bartimaeus (Mark 10.46f) vividly illustrates this aim of saving faith. Bartimaeus' faith is something much richer than mere faith in a healer; it's rather a faithful relation of dependence upon the Person of Christ. His cry is not "Thou Healer" but "Thou Son of David". He recognises Christ for what He really is. And Christ's words: "Thy faith hath made thee whole" are obviously charged with the same meaning that we have already noted regarding the one thankful leper. The "wholeness" is not of body only, but of personality. Hence, although Jesus need not be hindered in effecting a healing despite an inadequate level of faith on the part of the "patient", His aim and His desire was to see a man finding that deeper faith which illuminates the inner significance of the healing and makes it complete.

This distinction between "saving faith" and mere faith in the possibility of a healing was also valid for the Apostles. In the first few verses of the Book of Acts, chapter 3, we find Peter underlining the fact that it was "by faith in His name" that the man was made strong. "By faith in the name of Jesus, this man whom you see and know was made strong. It is Jesus' name and the faith that comes through Him that has given this complete healing to him, as you can all see" (N.I.V.).

Must we not, then, beware of being satisfied with a "faith" which looks only to "getting better", or a faith in Christ which is little more than a belief that His teachings are true? The faith with which we have to do is the faith that's of such a deeply personal nature that it remains unimpaired even when a physical healing doesn't take place.

Chapter 5

HEALING AND PERSONAL RELIGION (ii)

Perhaps enough has been said to underline the crucial point that, however a cure takes place, its permanence and its fullest benefit will be seen only where some change of inner attitude has taken place in the patient. Does this imply further that not only are illnesses the frequent product of certain attitudes of mind, but that by avoiding these attitudes altogether, such illnesses may never materialise? It does indeed — as modern psychosomatic medicine has already hinted.

Many people are reluctant to accept such a conclusion. It's much easier to believe that disease always arises outside the body and in a manner over which we have no control. The sober implications of accepting the idea that illness may originate in an unhealthy state of mind or soul are both obvious and embarrassing to many people. But, just as we can regret the attitude of the man who hopes to be cured without any effort of his own, we can also regret the attitude of the man who hopes to *avoid illness* without any effort of his own.

It is surely commonplace knowledge today that some illnesses are the inevitable result of certain negative emotions—which may suggest that private devotions could be not simply one method of healing sickness but a method of *preventing* such sickness. The relationship between health and personal religion is certainly one that's open to much fruitful exploring.

What, for example, might be the effects on health of an attitude of trustful composure? Most of us certainly know the negative effects of emotions like hate or resentment or worry or bad temper or jealousy. The author of the Book of Ecclesiasticus, in the Apocrypha, certainly knew all about it. "Jealousy and anger shorten life, and anxiety brings on old age too soon." Yes, the cause of many illnesses is to be found within ourselves. It's no mere extravagance of language to say that we often do "make ourselves sick". "As a man thinks in his heart, so is he." Negative emotions, if persisted in for a time, will frequently result in some physical or mental disharmony. Bertrand Russell may not have been a particularly religious man, but he was surely right when he wrote in *Authority and the Individual* that "We know too much and feel too little. At least we feel too little of those creative emotions from which a good life springs." Even more bluntly Joseph Roux, nearly a hundred years ago, claimed: "Nothing kills like the emotions". This is undoubtedly true of negative emotions.

It's widely acknowledged today that the abnormal tension, for example, under which many people live has been found to interfere with blood circulation to such an extent that the most common of all diseases are congestions of the blood, ending in inflammation. These, of course, are the illnesses whose medical names end with "itis". Their names are legion. Yet the cause can be basically the same in each case. The symptoms merely differ according to the particular tissue which is involved.

Most negative emotions like hate or anger or envy tend to result in tension, which inevitably prevents a free flow of blood since the muscles and fibres are considerably tightened up. Resultant inflammation won't disappear until the tension is relieved. This can be done in various ways, but the one that's not listed in the medical books is prayer! But prayer, as an expression of trustful composure, *can* do as much to relieve the physical condition as a material remedy, for prayer is — or can be — the expression of trustful composure, and it's just such an attitude which relieves the blood congestion and restores balance to the system once again. "O rest in the Lord" is now seen to be something more than a pious exhortation. It's one of the most practical bits of advice that any sick person can be offered.

Many doctors now acknowledge that negative emotions are the cause of many ulcers. Some years ago a survey revealed that, out of fifteen thousand ulcer patients, eighty per cent were found not to have any physical cause for ulcer of the stomach. Eight out of ten ulcers were caused by negative emotions or attitudes. Whether the ulcer be caused by too much hydrochloric acid being manufactured in the stomach, or by the failure of gland cells to manufacture enough gastric juice to break up the protein food, the same cause often applies to both — the effect of negative emotions on the body. In fact, not only do such emotions cause ulcers, but they can often be responsible for a relapse and for the recurrence of them.

In the light of this, perhaps the old evangelical appeal to "come to Jesus" is seen to have much more relevance to modern man's situation than he may have realised! "If you had only known the things which belong to your peace!" But, we repeat, religion must never be offered simply as a "remedy" for sickness. And yet, we mustn't go to the other extreme and play down this undeniably important "bonus" of Christian faith. A close relationship with Christ *does* help people to develop new and more positive thought-habits. It helps to replace every thought of fear with one of faith; every thought of illness with one of health; every thought of death with one of life. He helps people to throw off the sometimes "convenient" belief that their nature is something that cannot be altered. Surely religion has failed in one of its functions if a person's emotions aren't altered from negative to positive. The attitude of trustful composure is certainly one of the most powerful therapeutic influences available to us. "Let this mind be in you which was also in Christ Jesus."

But this attitude of trustful composure will be difficult to arrive at unless we are possessed by a deep awareness of the Love of God. Many patients do not possess it, and so healing, which flourishes best in an atmosphere of love, may be slow to take place. Certainly for the first few centuries of the Church's existence the sense of God's love for people was very real, and it was precisely when this sense of God's love was lost or diminished that attitudes to healing changed. Confidence in the possibility of healings decreased.

Now we believe that there are few situations more likely to cause mental and physical illness than a prolonged assurance in the mind of the patient that he is not loved. Many of the common neurotic complaints of modern civilisation have, significantly, been traced to this sense of uncertainty with regard to the Creator's love, as well as to unhappy experiences in childhood of unloving parents. Divine love isn't just a topic of conversation among Christians and of no concern to anyone else. It's a real stabilising and integrating power. Of course critics of Christianity find little meaning in such biblical statements as "God commends His love to us, in that, while we were still sinners, Christ died for us" (Rom.5.8). Perhaps they resent being called sinners, in the first place! Or perhaps they simply cannot imagine any love being powerful enough, and willing enough, to cancel out their faults. Either situation contains the seeds of mental, and therefore bodily, illness. It's the person who recognises the Love of God for what the Bible says it is who finds peace and harmony of soul, and who, therefore, is "favourably placed" as far as avoiding physical disharmony is concerned. The fact that Christians rarely go through life without *some* physical derangement doesn't make the principle invalid; for the question is still always open: What *more* serious and *more* frequent illnesses might he have suffered without the "balance" provided by a grateful acknowledgement of the Love of God?

Now, nobody would deny that constitutional factors play some part in the appearance of illness, and those who recommend healing through worship are fully aware of this. But it remains true that the man who does have a personal assurance of God's unconditional love is more favourably placed for all-round health than if he did not have that assurance. Such biblical statements as "perfect love casts out fear" have an intensely practical significance for us today; for, quite literally, love liberates people from many of their illnesses, because it liberates them from fear. Nothing is so vividly contrasted in the Gospel as the paralysing power of fear and the liberating power of love. "It is I," says Jesus; "be not afraid." There is, Christ makes clear, no single situation in life which is not transformed by the belief that "all things work together for good to those who love God". To know that in every situation, however critical or tragic it appears to be, God's love is shining through, is the most "therapeutic conviction" that we can hold. God's love is unconditional. Not only does that assurance "steady the nerves" as nothing—including drugs—can, but it also maintains the healthy rhythm of the body, as no external agency can.

There is a final point that we would like to make in this chapter in connection with healing and personal religion—and it concerns the healing power of forgiveness. The importance of divine forgiveness for a genuine religious experience has of course been maintained by all branches of the Christian Church since the beginning of Christianity—and by the Jewish tradition too. The Psalmist acknowledges not only that "there is forgiveness with Thee", but also that "blessed is he whose transgression is forgiven". The experience of such forgiveness was a vital ingredient in spiritual wellbeing. One wonders, however, whether the full blessedness of that experience is understood by many in the Church today. Some of them certainly regard forgiveness as exclusively a "religious category" — and we must, of course, not underrate the religious aspect of forgiveness. But perhaps the *medical* implications of forgiveness have been grossly under-emphasised.

The story of the Paralytic (Mark 2. 1-12) can shed a great deal of light on this topic. In it we find one of the best illustrations of the truth that physical illness can be cured by the creation of a new spiritual relationship to God. The curative factor in this "miracle" is the forgiveness of sins. The patient seems to have been suffering from a severe guilt-complex, which was broken up immediately the experience of divine forgiveness became real to him. This is by no means an unusual procedure, as many modern psychologists have confirmed. Paralysis *can* be caused by a sense of guilt, and it can also be cured by an acceptance of God's forgiveness. One of the oldest stories in the Bible — in the Book of Job — contains the belief that repressed guilt was a fruitful cause of illness; and, that this was the cause of the paralytic's illness was immediately seen by Jesus.

It may, of course, have been the unconscious part of the paralytic's mind which produced the illness; and it may even have been that it was produced so that, if his guilt were discovered, he would still be able to win sympathy. Some may call it a classic case of "conversion hysteria"—i.e. the conversion into physical terms of a mental state that has become intolerable. But, whereas the Rabbis had encouraged him to regard the illness as punishment, and had failed to speak of forgiveness, Christ dispelled both his fears and his guilt-complex by that assertion of forgiveness which affected not only his conscious mind, but also his unconscious—thus reaching the root of the sickness. When this was done, the physical illness was no longer "necessary"; nor was it appropriate to the newly gained health of mind and soul. Healing by an experience of divine forgiveness is certainly one of the most effective and seemingly miraculous methods of healing known to Christians today.

Unfortunately some people accept this kind of illness—or even *desire* it—as a kind of atonement for the guilt they feel. Some do so on a conscious level, others on the unconscious. But in either case a sort of satisfaction is obtained from the presence of the illness, and from the consequent "immunity from censure" which it secures for the patient. Even a complete breakdown in health, as doctors have told us, may be unconsciously desired in preference to the burden of facing up to some punishment which might follow the exposure of the sin. There is a well-documented story of a patient who, having committed a serious moral fault in the month of June, found each successive June that a dermatitis rash was set up, for no apparent reason. Only when the clear connection between his guilt and the rash was acknowledged—together with a humble acceptance of God's forgiveness—did the next June pass without any sign of the rash.

However, although a sense of God's forgiveness is one of the most powerful healing energies, it's essential to realise that this sense of forgiveness mustn't be regarded in the same light as some modern drug! Healing through worship—and this includes, of course, prayers of confession—is indeed a distinct possibility, but this is certainly not the main purpose of worship. To desire God's forgiveness simply because it has been found that a repressed guilt makes a man ill is a clear sign that the spiritual relationship between God and man is still faulty. Even a genuine sense of forgiveness, however, mustn't be taken to be the *guarantee* of a speedy physical recovery, such as was experienced by the Capernaum paralytic. The consequences of sin may often continue for a long time and may hold up a complete physical cure. But the point is that the necessary relationship has been established within which the maximum conditions for health of body and soul are created.

Psychology may sometimes help to bring guilt into full consciousness in a person, but the operative or curative factor in many a mental distress or physical derangement is to acknowledge that "in Christ" forgiveness is possible. As Burns once wrote of God,

"But Thou art good; and goodness still
Delighteth to forgive".

But unfortunately many a man believes in God without believing in His power, and His desire, to forgive sins. That kind of belief is likely to have a very limited effect on his religious life — and on his physical health.

The Christian religion will always have its element of "mystery", and there will always be some disagreement about certain aspects of its teaching. At the heart of its message, however, there surely is an offer of forgiveness which no one can misunderstand, though he may disbelieve or deride the very idea. And it's through the acceptance of this divine forgiveness that healing can so often occur.

"Plenteous grace with Thee is found,
Grace to cover all my sin;
Let the healing streams abound;
Make and keep me pure within."

In his book *A Faith to Proclaim*, that renowned Scottish preacher, James S. Stewart, wrote: "We are hearing much in these days about the Church and the ministry of healing. We are being told—I for one believe quite truly—that the Church has too much neglected this part of its commission. But there is one fact that is too often overlooked. It is this—that wherever the Church truly proclaims the forgiveness of sins, there the healing ministry is veritably at work. Who can tell the incalculable results of the word of absolution for the integration of human personalities? Who can say how much organic disease is being rooted out by the assurance of pardon and renewal?" May we not say that a very great deal is being rooted out in this way?

PART II

INTRODUCTION TO THE HEALING SERVICES

It is perhaps worth saying again that the method of *Healing Through Worship* is not intended to replace all other methods of healing. There are many channels through which we can receive God's healing power, and we believe each sick person has the responsibility of exploring as many of these channels as possible. But there is, we believe, no single channel of healing which isn't made more effective by regular devotion on the part of the patient. Even the most impersonal kind of treatment has a greater likelihood of doing maximum good when the relationship between the patient and his God is at its deepest and most personal.

There is an important reason why healing through worship should be regarded as a vital part of every person's healing. It reminds us as no other single healing method does, that a man's highest wellbeing comes through a conscious relationship to his Creator. What damage can be done, on occasion, by thinking of healing through prayer as a form of magic!

Certainly cures can be had, and they can be very spectacular, but readily the sickness may return if there is no positive readjustment to God. It's far better for a man to readjust to God *before* he is healed physically, than after—for, how easily man becomes "forgetful of all His benefits".

In fact, unless we are fully conscious of what is happening to us as we are being healed, there is often the danger of a relapse. That's why healing through mediums, or through hypnotism, or through highly emotional faith-healers can sometimes lead to profound disillusionment. As A.G. Ikin wrote in his *New Concepts of Healing*: "Methods that encourage personal responsibility and a direct responsiveness to the unseen, with ordinary consciousness undisturbed, make for greater stability and integration". Yet how many patients continue to hope against hope that this is not so, and that a purely impersonal, magical kind of healing is just as good?

Moreover, as we hinted in Part I, regular, private devotion doesn't merely offer a stronger possibility of becoming healed, but it can prevent illness altogether. None of us will ever attain to the spiritual perfection of Christ Himself, but it is at least suggestive that one of the reasons we never hear of Christ being ill is that he achieved perfect communion with His heavenly Father. Can most of us not acknowledge that some of our physical troubles—and perhaps mental ones too—may well arise from the fact that our communion with God is sporadic and imperfect? As Dr. Weatherhead commented in his *Psychology, Religion, and Healing*, "maximum health of spirit demands some form of worship, and worship, when it is true communion with God, has again and again proved to have won, as a by-product, increased health for the worshipper. Many who complain of their restlessness will fly to the doctor and the psychologist, when what they really hunger for is only to be found in God."

"The true basis of health is, in fact, spiritual," writes William Portsmouth in *Healing Prayer*. "Fullness of life begins with an inner relationship with the Giver of Life. It is by means of this relationship of spirit that the mind is informed with truth, and that the body, in turn, by its actions and reactions, reveals that truth physically." But we cannot argue people into that belief. All we can hope is that, if they persist in refuting the idea of worship as a pathway to prevention of illness, they may still, by the grace of God, find it to be a pathway to healing.

As to the Healing Services themselves, each one begins with the Lord's Prayer, which many generations of worshippers have found the best preparation for private devotion, and which should, where possible, be said aloud and spoken slowly, dwelling on each of the clauses in turn.

How better can we come into God's presence — or at least become aware of it — than by calling Him Father? And how better can we remind ourselves of His Purpose for us than by dwelling on the petitions that follow? Certainly we must believe, as we pray, that His name can be hallowed. that His kingdom can come, that His will can be done in our bodies as well as our souls. Then, isn't it a sign of spiritual health and genuine humility that we ask Him for daily bread? He isn't God of the soul only, but of the body too — and the two are, of course, intimately linked; for in one breath we ask for bread, and in the next forgiveness.

Then how often do we need to be "delivered from evil"? And who can do this better than our Lord? For His is indeed "the kingdom, the power, and the glory" — but He wants to share them with us, to use them for our benefit, to manifest them in us. Is this the kind of faith that we shall have consolidated in ourselves when the words of this perfect prayer have passed our lips?

We then turn to the reading of the Scriptures — in each case one of the Gospel healings performed by Jesus. As we read, perhaps we should remember why these stories appear in written form at all. They were written down not merely to show Jesus as a wonder-

42

worker, but to evoke the faith of those who read them. And how can these verbal pictures of compassion and love do anything other than that? But, of course, they do more. They give us a real cause for hope, as far as our own cure is concerned. In each story we see that God's will for His people is health, and that sickness is an invasion upon the natural order. Each story reminds us that God doesn't *need* illness to achieve His purpose, and that He certainly does not *send* illness as a punishment. As we read, let's endeavour in the imagination to put ourselves in the position of those whom Jesus cured, and believe fervently in His power to heal.

There then follows a short devotional comment on the Bible passage, not merely to help us understand it a little better, but to focus its message of comfort and challenge and to help us see it as a pointer to our own possible healing. As the approximate number of Gospel healings is twenty-five, these 25 Healing Services thus form a kind of short devotional commentary on the cures performed by Jesus.

This naturally leads on to prayer. While the prayers set down in Part II may well express the thoughts of most worshippers, some of the prayers might, of course, be replaced by "spontaneous" ones if so desired. But again it is recommended that the prayers should be spoken aloud, and slowly. It's not essential, of course, for all the prayers to be used on the one occasion.

Any who intend using these Healing Services, but who find them slightly long, or who find it difficult to concentrate, may wish to omit the meditation. But it is hoped that normally these Services would provide a well-balanced form for private devotion, lasting ten minutes or so.

FIRST HEALING SERVICE

The Lord's Prayer

The Bible Reading

"Leaving that place, He withdrew to the neighbourhood of Tyre, and, wishing to remain unrecognised, shut Himself up indoors. But He did not succeed in hiding Himself. A woman whose daughter had an unclean spirit heard about Him at once, and came and cast herself at His feet. She was a Greek, of Syrophoenician descent. She asked Him repeatedly to cast the demon out of her daughter.

'First let the children have their fill', he said to her; 'for it is not right to take the children's bread and throw it to the house-dogs.' She took this up and said: 'True, Lord; yet the house-dogs under the table *do* feed — on the children's crumbs'.

He said to her: 'Thanks to that saying you may go in peace. The demon has come out of your daughter.' And the woman went home and found her child laid on the bed, and the demon gone." (Mark, ch. 7)

The Meditation

Here's a story which many students of the Bible regard as one of the most difficult in

Mark's Gospel. Yet it has a word for us that's clear and striking. To start with, isn't it a cause for gratitude that Christ *likes* to fail in His attempt to hide Himself? He likes to be sought and found. He likes people to go to the trouble of looking for Him. For, this is a sign not just of need, but of faith. One question, therefore, that we might ask ourselves is this: "Have we been put off by the fact that God's help seems difficult to find?"

Another question is this: "Have we, like this woman, asked Christ *repeatedly* to minister to our infirmity—or have we stopped asking in face of His seeming reluctance to do anything for us?" It's a sober thought that, had this woman interpreted Christ's seeming indifference to her cry as final, her little daughter might never have been healed. Am *I* guilty of thinking Christ's apparent "No" to my first request means a "No" to all others? Many a sufferer has condemned *himself* to continued illness simply because of this attitude.

Is it right that I should understand Christ's seemingly severe words to this woman as a way of testing her? It certainly is! He's pointing out that His gospel of "wholeness" is, in the first place, for the Jew, not the Gentile; and, of course, many a woman would have seen that as a firmly shut door. But not this woman of faith. She was perfectly willing to take the "left-overs"; and that, so she believed, would be more than enough. Here, in this story, I have the "proof" that no one, saint or sinner, churchman or non-churchman, is denied an answer to genuine faith.

Here, indeed, was a woman who believed in the possibility of "absent healing". Can *I* not believe in the possibility of *present* healing? One thing is sure: He longs to say to me, "You may go in peace".

My Prayer for Today

Lord Christ, my Saviour, hear me today as I bring my need before You, and help me to that reverence and awe of You which is the beginning of knowledge. May I know my need not just of bodily healing, but also of the healing of the soul. May I know You not just as Redeemer of my sickness, but also Redeemer of my sin. May I know You not just as a God whom I can use, but as a God who desires to use me.

If I have drawn a veil across Your glory by my persistent unbelief and blindness, grant me peace, O Lord, and a new vision of You.

If I have clouded over the Divine Light by my tendency to despair and to fear, grant me patience, O Lord, and a new trust in You.

If I have frustrated Your purpose of wholeness by my pessimism and lack of persistence, grant me power, O Lord, and a new zeal for You.

I pray You, Father of all, to bless all those of

47

my fellow-sufferers who still seek relief at Your hand. Preserve them from the temptation of accepting their illness as Your will. Help them to see that nothing may hinder their wholeness except their too-ready submission and their too-slow cooperation.

> O Physician of men, give the grace of wisdom to all doctors.
>
> O Sanctifier of men, give the grace of holiness to all ministers of Your Word.
>
> O Lover of men, give the grace of tenderness to all who watch over the sick.

For Jesus' sake.　Amen

SECOND HEALING SERVICE

The Lord's Prayer
The Bible Reading

"On a Sabbath day, when He was teaching in one of the synagogues, a woman appeared who had been possessed by an infirmity for eighteen years. She was bent double and quite unable to lift up her head. When Jesus saw her, He called her to Him and said: 'Woman, you are rid of your infirmity'; and He laid His hands on her.

She was made straight immediately and praised God. But the governor of the synagogue took the matter up. He was indignant because Jesus had healed on the Sabbath, and he said to the congregation: 'There are six days when it is right for us to work. Come and be healed on one of them, and not on the Sabbath day.'

'You hypocrites', the Lord replied to this. 'On the Sabbath do you not one and all loose your ox or donkey from the manger and take him off to water him? And this woman, this daughter of Abraham, whom Satan bound, yes, eighteen years ago—was it not right for her to have been loosed from those bonds of hers on the Sabbath day?'

When He said this, all His antagonists were

put to shame, and the people thought with joy of all the glorious things that He was doing." (Luke 13)

The Meditation

Jesus has nothing whatever in common with those who, for religious or other scruples, would postpone healing to a "more suitable moment". *Now* is the day of salvation. Maybe I even feel that I'm not worthy to be healed at the moment and am not therefore making much effort to claim His own promise to me. Maybe I feel— perhaps subconsciously—that my sickness is a punishment from God for something I have done, or not done, and so I'm not taking seriously Christ's power to heal me.

Well, however I may try to explain away this woman's trouble, there's no denying the wonder of this healing of somebody who had been bent double for eighteen years. I don't know how it happened but I know it did—and that it can happen again today. Just because I haven't been made straight at once, I know I mustn't doubt or despair, for God heals in the way He thinks best, and I believe that way *is* best.

Here, certainly, is a straight answer to those who deceive themselves with the idea that their illness is the will of God. Illness is to be fought and overcome. But even God needs, and desires, our help; *my* help. This woman helped her *total* healing (i.e. of mind and soul as well as body) by praising God. Have I helped Him by giving thanks for the least sign of improvement? For thankfulness is one small key to wholeness. I know it, but how difficult I find it to put it into effect in my prayers!

The question this story leaves with me seems to be this: do I want wholeness *merely* to be rid of my discomfort, or so that I might the more be able to glorify God? My answer to that, I know, is bound to affect the possibility of a cure. Must I not then think with joy of all the great things He can do, *and* of the glorious Being that He is in Himself?

My Prayer for Today

O Lord, You who hear my prayers and answer them — even though it may not always be the answer I want — grant me a fresh measure of faith as I pray now.

O Lord, You who love my soul and sustain it — even though I'm hardly aware of the fact — grant me a new sensitiveness to the holy presence of Your life-giving Spirit.

O Lord, You who offer me pardon and can bestow it — even though I grieve You constantly by my self-assurance — grant me a new and lively sense of my dependence on You for all I am and have.

I pray today for those who help you in the sacred task of ridding people of their infirmities; for those who have been brought to a richer knowledge of You through their healing of body; for those who find it difficult to believe in Your healing purpose. (*Silent prayer*) Be with the sad and the sorrowful, with the lonely and the unloved, with the disillusioned and the despairing—and may Your healing light shine into the darkness of their lives, bringing pardon and peace.

You love me, Saviour Christ: may I love You.

You live in me, Blessed Spirit: may I live in You.

You listen to me, my Father: may I listen to You. Amen.

THIRD HEALING SERVICE

The Lord's Prayer
The Bible Reading

"As He passed along, He saw a man who had been blind from birth. His disciples put a question to Him. 'Rabbi,' they said, 'when this man was born blind, was it he or his parents that had sinned?'

Jesus replied: 'Neither he nor his parents had sinned. What was desired was that through this man the way in which God works should be made manifest.' With that, He spat on the ground, made clay with the spittle and smeared it on the man's eyes. Then He said: 'Go now and wash yourself in the Pool of Siloam'.

The man went and washed himself, and when he came away he could see. His neighbours said: 'Isn't this the man who sits and begs?' Some said it was. Others said no, though they saw a likeness. Meanwhile the man himself kept saying it was he. So they said to him: 'if that is true, how were your eyes opened?' And he replied: 'The man called Jesus made clay, smeared it on my eyes and told me to go to Siloam and wash. I went and washed myself, and I could see' " (John 9).

The Meditation

Here's a story that touches us all. For, aren't we all prompted to ask the question which has been asked for many centuries: "Where does sin come from?" and the further question: "Is my illness the result of sins I've committed?" Christ's questioners didn't doubt for a moment that *somebody* had sinned. They took it for granted that this man's affliction was somebody's fault.

Christ's answer is authoritative — and comforting. "Neither he nor his parents had sinned." In a word, a man's illness is *not* a punishment for sin. Yet, how often have I heard someone say to me: "What have I done to deserve this?" In most cases the answer is probably "nothing". Here, then, is something for me to ponder: have *I* got rid of that Old Testament notion about illness being *inevitably* bound up with sin?

Of course some illness *is* intimately connected with sin. Not as a punishment from God, but perhaps the unavoidable outcome of wrong living. Perhaps I have inflicted my present illness on myself by over-indulgence or by refusing to take my sense of guilt to Jesus for forgiveness — in which case this is self-punishment! If I cherish a grudge and this produces an ulcer, this is surely not a punishment from God!

But, however an illness is caused, the truth stands: that Christ is desirous, and is able, to cure it — usually with some sort of cooperation from the sufferer, as in this Bible story. The truth also stands that, from one point of view, even *my* illness, like the blind man's, is upon me so that the "way in which God works should be made manifest". This is a bold way of looking at suffering, but how much more sensible it is than believing suffering is inflicted on me by a revengeful God!

My Prayer for Today

Lord Christ, I come to You with my affliction today, believing You are ready to take it away. But grant, O Lord, that I may not be asking for healing of body when my soul is not at peace; that I may not be hoping for relief when my sin remains unconfessed and unforgiven; that I may not be expecting You to do everything when I have done nothing.

O Prince of Peace, I claim Your gift of a tranquil heart, by faith in You!

O Provider of Pardon, I claim Your gift of forgiveness, by faith in You!

O Promiser of Power, I claim Your gift of strength, by faith in You!

Often I have been fearful as well as ignorant, and often I have been weak as well as cynical. Gracious Lord, put a new spirit within me, preserving my soul from shrinking under adversity, and saving me from the false piety of *over*-ready submission to Your supposed will. Save me too, good Lord, from becoming morbid over my constant failures in love, and help me to seek the forgiveness which can set me on the right road again.

Certainly I have not had the faith I should have had. But if I have it now, I know You must have forgiven me. Bring that faith to full flower, Lord Jesus, through the daily devotion which I offer You. For Your name's sake.

Amen.

FOURTH HEALING SERVICE

The Lord's Prayer

The Bible Reading

"After this the Lord appointed others, seventy in number, and despatched them ahead of Him in pairs to every town and place that He Himself intended to visit . . . When you come to a town where they make you welcome, eat what is put before you, heal their sick, and say 'The Kingdom of God has approached you'.

The Seventy came back to Him rejoicing. 'Lord,' they said, 'the use of your name brings the very demons under our control' " (Luke 10).

The Meditation

It's strange how some people can still claim that healing was only a sideline in the disciples' ministry! But is it any less strange that there are those who regard the possibility of a personal healing through non-medical channels as very remote indeed? Perhaps *I* am one of such a group. If so, mustn't I rediscover the vital connection between wholeness and worship? Mustn't I rediscover that, by accepting the Word preached by these faithful disciples, and still preached today, I am a long way towards finding myself healed? Yes, in body as well as in soul?

What may I not expect or hope for by worshipping my Saviour here, in the privacy of my home or my bed? Mightn't I, for instance, find that my heart has opened itself to God's forgiveness, and that this was all I needed to be cured of my functional illness? Might I not even find a new and more real experience of His love for me, and so become free from those inner tensions and stresses which are prolonging, or even causing, my *organic* trouble?

It's fascinating to read that these disciples, who at first must have been a little hesitant at the very idea of healing in Jesus' name, returned to report that even "demons" were subject to His name. In other words, not even the most serious trouble known to man is outside the sway of Christ's power to heal. We today mightn't use the word "demon" to explain men's troubles, yet are we really much wiser today about the *ultimate* origin of people's worst afflictions? It's as true today as in the early years of the Church that the healing power of Christ avails "for all thy diseases". It avails for mine.

In this story the disciples are really reminding me that it's quite possible I may, through the use of the Lord's name, be able to bring my personal "demon" under control. How seriously have I thought of this possibility?

My Prayer for Today

O Lord Christ, the Healer of men's sicknesses, I ask Your forgiveness for putting limits on Your power, and I ask for Your strength for the renewal of faith within my heart, that I may earnestly believe that "*all* things are possible with You". O Lord, the demons of fear and despair are threatening to destroy me; deliver me, Saviour Christ! The demons of pain and distress are threatening to subvert my desire to live; deliver me, Saviour Christ!

Help me, gracious Father, to know that perfect health is Your will for me, and for all Your children; and grant that nothing may hinder those prayers of mine which may well be part of the channel along which Your healing power can come.

Bless the work of healing going on in the world, whether it be the preaching of Your Word, the treatment of men's minds, or the doctoring of their bodies; whether it be by medical treatment, or by cheering the sick or by the simple prayer of faith — for You, Lord, are the power behind all healing, and I give the glory to You alone.

Eternal God, You are Almighty, and I believe Your power can heal me.

Eternal God, You are All-wise, and I believe You will heal me how and when You deem best.

Eternal God, You are All-good, and I believe Your favour is never withheld from me in sickness or in health.

For my friends and acquaintances who are ill, I pray today, Father. (*Silent prayer*) Be with those confined to bed, and give them the promise and hope of walking again. Be with those in constant pain, and give them the promise and hope of liberty and peace. Be with those whose bodies are ill through disharmony of soul and give them the promise and hope of divine pardon and renewal of spirit.   Amen.

FIFTH HEALING SERVICE

The Lord's Prayer
The Bible Reading

"By the sheep-gate in that city (Jerusalem) there is a pool with five arcades. A number of disabled people, blind, lame, and withered used to lie in these arcades; and there was a man there who had suffered from his trouble for thirty-eight years.

Jesus, seeing him lying there and knowing that he had been ill for a long time, said to him: 'Have you the will to become well again?' 'Sir,' said the sick man, 'I have no one to put me in the pool when the water is ruffled, and while I am on the way someone else gets in before me.'

Jesus said: 'Rise, pick up your stretcher and walk'. And immediately the man was cured, picked up his stretcher and walked. Later, Jesus came upon him in the Temple and said: 'See now, you have been cured. Sin no more, lest something worse happen to you' " (John 5).

The Meditation

Is it credible that anyone who *really* wanted to get into the Pool with Five Arcades should have failed to do so, year after year, for thirty-eight years! Jesus clearly thought that this man hadn't tried very hard. "Have you the will to become well again?" A strange question indeed – unless He was quite certain the man *didn't* have the will to become well again.

Here is a very sober truth—one which explains a surprising number of "failures" in the realm of healing by faith. Illness is, let's admit it, a means of escape sometime from the necessity of facing up to life. Many is the patient today who scolds the healer for inefficiency, when the real trouble is that he himself doesn't actually want to be cured.

Mustn't I at least ask myself whether I don't get a certain amount of sympathy and limelight in being ill, which I'm unwilling to give up? The answer probably is that this doesn't apply to me—but there's no harm in asking the question—just in case! For there's a warning in this story even for me, and a reminder that my expressed wish to be healed *need* not correspond with my real feelings in the matter. Mustn't I examine my heart to see if, deep down, I do find it easier to face my physical handicaps than the heavy demands which life would make upon me if I were well?

I think of the well-known story of a lady whose illness had been diagnosed as inoperable cancer. Later she was told the doctors had made a mistake, and that she was completely free of the disease. But, instead of receiving the news with joy — the normal reaction, surely! — she received it almost with resentment. To be told she was in good health was actually a bigger blow than to be told she was going to die! Her own comment is revealing: "I cannot bear the thought of facing life again".

Maybe I'm not a confirmed neurotic like the man of Bethesda, but if I took Jesus at His word, could I too not "rise . . . and walk"? Maybe I haven't exactly run away from life, but maybe I have lost the vision of a full and healthy life and so have lost not just hope for myself, but faith in Christ.

It seems that Jesus caught this man's attitude just in time. For, if he had "sinned more", i.e. continued in his cowardly attitude to life, a worse thing might have happened to him — perhaps an even worse neurosis. *Not* that Jesus blamed him or castigated him, but how could He view this man's spiritual plight with unconcern?

And He's deeply concerned about mine. He doesn't censure me when He says "Sin no more", but I have to admit that I have committed the sin of unbelief, the sin of *too* ready submission, the sin of wanting things done the easy way. But He wants my faith; and He needs my intelligent cooperation if my healing is to be of soul as well as body. How badly do I want to give these things to Him — now?

My Prayer for Today

O You who are the strength of my life, forgive me that I've been so weak.

O You who are the hope of my life, forgive me that I've so easily despaired.

O You who are the goal of my life, forgive me that I've rested content with lesser things.

Gracious Lord, I have suffered much, but I praise you that You have preserved within my soul the genuine desire to get well. I have prayed much and praise You for the patience you have given me to "continue instant in prayer", though little seems to happen to me. I've seen others getting well before me, but You have graciously kept me from bitterness and from the temptation to make my illness an escape from life. Praise be to You, O God!

Yet grant to me, loving Spirit, that I might listen even more carefully to the voice of the Eternal, my God; that I might pay even greater heed to Your commands; that I might be enabled to follow all Your rules, and so find the health that's normal for true Christian manhood. Help me to regard sickness as an intrusion into Your lovely world. Help me to regard suffering as an evil which Christ came to conquer. And though You can often use it to fashion saintliness, preserve me from thinking that sickness is essential to Your purpose.

You, Father, see me whole again. May my faith in You and my will to live help speed my salvation. You, Father, see me as one re-created in Your image. May it not be that my faults or my fears might frustrate that purpose of Yours. For Jesus' sake.   Amen.

SIXTH HEALING SERVICE

The Lord's Prayer

The Bible Reading

"Now one of the noblemen at court had a son lying sick at Capernaum. Hearing that Jesus had moved from Judaea into Galilee, this man sought Him out and begged Him to come down from Cana and cure his son, who was at the point of death. Jesus said: 'Will nothing but the sight of miracles and portents make you believe?' 'Sir,' said the nobleman, 'come down before my child is dead.' 'You can go back', said Jesus. 'Your son is living.' And the man set out, convinced that he had heard the truth from Jesus.

As he was travelling down, he was met by his servants with the news that his boy was living, and he asked them when he had got better. 'The fever left him yesterday,' they said, 'at noon.' Then the father realised that this had happened at the very time when Jesus said to him: 'Your son is living'. And he and his whole family believed" (John 4).

The Meditation

This account reads very much like the story of the Centurion's servant, but the present story is distinctive enough to bring a special message of comfort—and of challenge—to me. How fervent, in the first place, was this distracted father's cry to the Saviour of men! His willingness to seek Jesus out instead of vaguely hoping that He *might* come and do something is a lesson in itself. For, have I sought Him out anxiously enough: in prayer, for instance? or in the Bible? or in the ministrations of my doctor or minister? For He's there, in every case, just waiting to yield to the persistence of faith.

Christ's first reaction to the nobleman is perhaps easy to understand, for He had been thronged by people who had little other motive for attending to Him than the hope to see Him do something really sensational. "Will nothing but the sight of miracles and portents make you believe?" Certainly that's all that some people seem to care about.

Well, the stricken father didn't stop to argue with Jesus. But he made it perfectly plain that his love for his son was far greater than his desire for a mere miracle for miracle's sake. And that's all Jesus wanted to know. "You can go back. Your son is living." That's exactly what Christ says to me when He sees my love to be greater than my curiosity. When I request help for my illness, if He sees that I have even the makings of faith in His power to heal, as distinct from the mere desire to see a miracle done in me, He's only too ready to help me.

And yet, when He does speak the word, promising me healing, do I always "set out, convinced that I have heard the truth from Jesus?" This man did, and what a wonderful fulfilment of faith was waiting for him when he arrived home! Is it so very remarkable that this man's son began to get better from the moment Jesus spoke the word? Haven't millions of people begun to get better when the Word of God found an entrance into their hearts? The really important question for me seems to be this: Do I genuinely believe that I can begin to get better, in body *and* in soul, when I hear the word of promise and power spoken to my heart?

My Prayer for Today

Lord Christ, who are present in all places and yet unknown to so many people, I rejoice today that You are ever ready to hear the prayer of faith.

Teach me, gracious Saviour, to lay all my troubles before You, knowing that, until I do so, You may not be able to help me.

Teach me, gracious Sustainer, to trust myself more readily and more lovingly to Your care, and so find that my trust leads to Your peace.

Teach me, gracious Sovereign, to dedicate my will more zealously to Yours, and so enter that service which is perfect freedom.

In the light of Your love for men who are loveless, I adore You today.

In the light of Your faith in men who are faithless, I adore You, O Christ.

In the light of Your Promise towards men whose lives seem almost without promise, I adore You, O my God.

Grant that my adoration may not be marred by petitions which would shame Your purpose. Grant that my desires and delights may be in accordance with Your will. And grant that my sufferings and my sighings may never hide You from me.

Prosper your own sacred work of healing not just in me but in the whole company of those who are bound together in the fellowship of infirmity. Hear my prayer for those whom I especially love and whose names I bring lovingly before You. (*Silent prayer*) Bless them each one, Father.   Amen.

SEVENTH HEALING SERVICE

The Lord's Prayer
The Bible Reading

"They came to Bethsaida, and the people brought Him a blind man and besought Him to touch him. He took the blind man by the hand and led him out of the village. Then, after spitting on his eyes and laying His hands on him, He asked: 'Can you distinguish anything?' The man looked up and said: 'I can distinguish the men, for I see them like trees, walking about'.

He then put His hands once more on the eyes and the man saw clearly. His sight had been restored and he could now distinguish even distant objects well" (Mark 8).

The Meditation

So many of Christ's miracles of healing have to do with the restoring of sight to the blind, and most of them are recorded two or three times in the different gospels. But here is one which we find nowhere except in St. Mark. Is this coincidence, I wonder? Probably not; for, whereas in the other healings of blindness Christ restores His patients' sight at once, here it is done in stages; and all of the other gospel writers (who, of course, wrote *after* Mark) may have thought it inadvisable to include it in case it suggested any insult to Christ's power. If this is so, what a pity. For is it really any less marvellous that a man should be cured gradually than immediately? *I* may be one who is tempted to think so.

As far as the blind man of our story is concerned, it's quite possible Jesus was influenced by the fact that the glare of the Eastern sun might have damaged the eyes again if the cure had been immediate—in which case the story certainly pinpoints His wisdom as well as His power. The question *I* might ask myself here is this: if I were cured suddenly, is it possible there might be loss as well as gain? Maybe not. But maybe I would be spiritually unprepared for a sudden bodily healing, and would use my cure for selfish purposes; whereas by the spiritual discipline of regular prayer I am more likely to secure a healing which will be used to the greater glory of God. The possibility is at least worth considering.

One thing I do note for my comfort—something much more important than the question as to why Jesus used saliva—namely, the fact that He aimed at a complete cure. He doesn't do things by half-measures. And yet so many people think their partial cure is the most they can expect and the most they're going to get, which may sometimes frustrate Christ in His desire to complete it. Let me see to it that I don't do that! Christ wills me to be whole; but do I really want to be?

My Prayer for Today

O Lord Jesus Christ, Your ways are often mysterious, yet Your will is perfectly plain. Your power is often unfelt, yet Your promises shine forth as the stars. Your likeness in me is often effaced, yet Your love is always directed my way.

Help me, Saviour, to be more trusting in Your wisdom, anticipating only that which is good. Help me to hope even when there seems to be no help. And grant that I may surrender to You every unworthy thought and every damaging emotion.

There are many of my friends, O God, who bring me before You in prayer and ask You to touch me. Some of them wish me to be cured as earnestly as I do. Open my heart, Lord, to the atmosphere of that love. Grant even that it may serve as the oil of Your healing power; and may my own selflessness and devotion further invite the presence of that same power.

O Light of men's bodies, shine even now into the fibres of my flesh and open the windows of my soul to Your rays.

O Truth of men's minds, present Yourself with power to the eyes of my understanding, and may I accept it with joy.

O End of men's souls, make me more and more sensitive to Your perfect holiness, that I may see Your kingdom as my goal.

Open my eyes, Father of all mankind, to the many different needs of Your suffering people. Help me to see that my prayers for myself are of greatest avail when I have prayed also for others. So take my requests now as a genuine expression of my love for those whom I name in the silence of my heart. Make them whole — and make me whole — O Christ my Lord.   Amen.

EIGHTH HEALING
SERVICE

The Lord's Prayer

The Bible Reading

"They came to the Gerasenes' country on the far side of the Sea, and He had no sooner disembarked than a man with an unclean spirit came out from the tombs and confronted him. This man lived in the sepulchres and had reached a stage when no one could control him, even by the use of chains. Now, seeing Jesus from afar, he ran up, fell at His feet and cried with a loud voice: 'What is your business with me, Jesus, Son of God the highest? I adjure you by God not to torment me.' (For Jesus had been saying to him: 'Unclean spirit, come out of that man'.)

'What is your name?' Jesus asked him. 'My name is legion,' he replied; 'for there are many of us.' There was a large herd of pigs feeding on the mountainside, and the spirits begged Him to send them among the pigs. He gave them leave, and the unclean spirits came out and entered the pigs, with the result that the herd charged down the cliff into the sea.

Their herdsmen fled and brought the news to

the town and countryside; and the people approached Jesus and saw the demoniac sitting there, dressed and in his right mind — the very man who had had the legion in him. As Jesus was stepping into the boat, the man who had been possessed begged Him to let him stay with Him. But Jesus said to him: 'Go home now to your own people, and tell them what great things the Lord God has done for you, and the mercy He showed you' " (Mark 5).

The Meditation

This story, better than any other in the New Testament, shows how false it is to claim that Jesus never bothered to find out the exact nature of the troubles He cured. He suited His technique to the patient. He refused, in *this* case, simply to lay hands on him and put all the responsibility of being cured on the patient himself. Jesus cures always by the most appropriate method, the one which offers the best guarantee of a permanent cure — for even His healings can be undone through man's lack of cooperation.

Many a trouble can be healed by suggestion — and Christ sometimes uses this method. But when He tried it on this demented man, it was clear he hadn't the necessary personal relationship with the Healer — the relationship without which suggestion is fruitless. And so, after spending half the night with him (doing what doctors might call "diagnosing"), Christ gets the man to see that his whole personality is shot through by conflicting interests and drives—which is what the Bible means by "unclean spirits".

The actual story of *how* the unclean spirits were driven out is unimportant compared with the simple fact that they *were* driven out. The ex-demoniac was found by a very surprised group of people to be "sitting there, and in his right mind". This may be a picture not too remote from my own experience! For, though I may not suffer from split-personality, don't I recognise that my personality is far from being whole? And don't I know in my heart that this spiritual disharmony and dispeace has no small effect upon my physical trouble?

This much I know, that the Christ who heals the mind is the same Christ who heals the body. And if I let Him possess me, there's little chance that evil will possess either my body or my mind. How fervently am I begging Him now to "send my unclean spirits among the pigs"?

My Prayer for Today

O Saviour Christ, who have compassion upon men's sicknesses of body, mind, and soul, I acknowledge today that I am whole in no part of me. Grant me, Lord, relief for the pains of my body, resolution for the discords of my mind, and refreshment for the aridness of my

76

soul. And make me alive, O God, not just to the possibility of healing, but also to the healing power itself.

O Perfect Holiness, forgive and cast out all that is coarse and unclean in me.

O Perfect Humanity, forgive and cast out all that is mean and carnal in me.

O Perfect Health, forgive and cast out all that is evil and incomplete in me.

I pray today for those of my fellow-sufferers who are grievously ill in their minds; for those without the kindly light of reason, that they may soon "sit there, dressed, and in their right minds"; for those who have become perverted in their thinking, that they may soon find the Truth which sets men free; for those who lie in mental homes, that they may understand at least something of Your peace.   Amen.

NINTH HEALING SERVICE

The Lord's Prayer

The Bible Reading

"One day Jesus was teaching, and in full possession of the healing power of God, when some men arrived, carrying on a couch a paralytic whom they wanted to bring in and lay down before Him. But the house was so packed with people that they couldn't see a way to get him in. So they went up on the roof and through the tiles let him down into the middle of the gathering, couch and all, at Jesus' feet.

Seeing their faith, Jesus said: 'Man, your sins have been forgiven you'. The doctors of the Law and the Pharisees began to turn this over in their minds. 'Who is this blaspheming?' they said. 'Who can forgive sins but God alone?' Jesus, aware of their thoughts, said: 'What are you thinking to yourselves? Which is the easier thing, to say "Your sins have been forgiven you"or to say "Get up and walk"? However, to teach you that the Son of Man has authority on earth to forgive sins'—and He turned to the paralysed man—'I say to you, Get up, take your couch, and walk home'.

The man rose immediately in view of the

people, picked up the couch he had been lying on, and went home praising God. They were all dumbfounded and praised God in their awe. 'We never thought', they said, 'to see what we have seen today' " (Luke 5).

The Meditation

How eloquent this story is, of Christ's power not only over sickness, but also over sin! Why, I wonder, did the evangelist write this story down? Was he more interested in the physical miracle than anything else? I hardly think so. St. Luke tells me this story now so that I might believe not just in the possibility of a physical cure, but also in Christ's authority to forgive those sins in me which *may* be hindering that cure.

Here was a man who became cured because he had been brought into a new spiritual relationship with the Lord of life. It was as easy — or as difficult — as that. The curative factor was the forgiveness of sins. And how often that's the case. There are thousands today who might get up and walk if they could only believe in, and accept, the forgiveness of sin so freely offered in His Word. Nothing is more important in healing through worship than the claiming of this forgiveness. Have *I* done just that?

There are those who ridicule the very idea that this Man of Nazareth has power to forgive sin. These are the same people who ridicule the

79

idea that He has the power to heal a man by non-physical means. Yet He does forgive today, and He does heal today! The two operations are really one. Maybe I don't disbelieve His power to forgive sin but am still hesitant about His forgiving *mine*. Maybe I'm conscious of some unforgiven sin. Maybe my sense of guilt has caused paralysis—of spirit or mind, if not of body. It's even possible that, like this man, I have some "complex" which has seeped right through into my unconscious mind. It's even possible that my illness relieves me of the necessity of facing up to my guilt.

If so, should I not, and can I not, tune my ears to the voice which is whispering now: "Man, your sins have been forgiven you"? For, if I do this, may I not find that I too will be able to get up, take my couch, and walk home?

My Prayer for Today

Lord Christ, my guilt is small compared with Your glory; my faults are trivial compared with Your forgiveness; my straits fade into insignificance beside Your strength. Yet, if I don't honestly recognise my weakness, I may still remain unaware of Your power. So grant me courage, O Lord, to see and deplore the worst in myself, but preserve me from failing to see and adore the Best in You. Cast out all my faulty reactions to life, my foolish resistance to love, my faithless refusal of liberty, and open

80

the doors of my heart to receive Your healing Spirit!

I feel You dwelling within me, Spirit of Life — even though I am preventing You from doing the great work which is Your goal. For the way in which the love and prayers of others have winged Your love towards me, I rejoice today. For the great fellowship of devotion throughout the world, I thank You, Father. For the faithful labour of physicians and nurses and all those dedicated to the cause of healing, I offer You my praise.

I have often been forgetful of Your Promises, O God; but I know in my heart that "the prayer of faith will restore the sick man, and that the Lord will raise him up". Help me to claim that promise for myself, now. I know, O God, that even the sins I have committed will be forgiven me. Help me to claim that promise for myself, now.

Let me not desire good for myself without desiring it also for others. Let Your blessing rest upon me and upon all others who know that nothing will separate them from Your love which is in Christ Jesus our Lord.　　　Amen.

TENTH HEALING SERVICE

The Lord's Prayer

The Bible Reading

"During His stay in one of the cities, there suddenly appeared a man who was covered with leprosy. When he saw Jesus he prostrated himself in supplication. 'Lord,' he said, 'if You will, you can cleanse me.' Jesus stretched out His hand, touched him, and said: 'I will it. Be cleansed.' And the leprosy left him immediately.

Jesus ordered him to tell no one. 'But go and show yourself to the priest,' He said, 'and make the offering for your purification which Moses prescribed, so that the people might be notified.' Yet Jesus' fame was more than ever blazed abroad, and large crowds gathered to hear Him and to be cured of their infirmities" (Luke 5).

The Meditation

The phrase "prostrated himself" is certainly significant! Here was a man who had the right spirit about being healed. No half-measures; no feelings that he *deserved* to be healed; no wrong ideas about leaving everything to Christ.

First, this man *worshipped*; and who can deny that this is the ideal preliminary to healing? And it's clear how powerfully this man's worship was charged with faith. "Lord, if you will, you can cleanse me." Is that my attitude too? or is my worship charged with doubt? I remember that it has been amply shown in reports of non-physical healing that a big percentage of cures have taken place largely through the nourishing of a genuine desire to get well. Just how genuinely do *I* desire to get well?

Certainly Christ's response to the leper's worshipful attitude was typical—and encouraging. "I will it; be cleansed." Yes, healed with a word. Does this seem rather fantastic? Surely not; for it happens often today. People with a sense of injustice frequently develop skin troubles— troubles which disappear immediately this attitude is changed. Didn't Job develop a skin disease after the shock of losing his material possessions? and the first step to healing is the same today as then: worship. "He prostrated himself."

My Prayer for Today

Lord Christ, who can heal with a word, I feel almost an outcast from the normal life of the world, and I ask You to cleanse me. You know the sadness of pain and affliction; indeed You are bearing some of my sorrow now. Grant that

83

I may not hinder the healing You are waiting to work within me by doubt or fear or blatant unbelief.

I would pray, Lord, not just for the continuing of Your healing power in me, but also in others. Be with the sick in mind or body or soul. Be with those who feel their ailment makes them exiles from the love of their fellows, and give them to know that You not only will their health, but can indeed make them clean. Prosper the ministrations of doctors and nurses, and bless the prayers of the faithful wherever they may be. (*Silent prayer*)

Today, Lord, You have given me grace to endure and to hope.

Today, Lord, You have moved within me and touched my heart.

Today, Lord, You have helped me to trust and to pray.

Grant that in the days to come I may have patience and courage and faith, and find the fulfilment of Your promise to heal drawing nearer and nearer. In all the worship of my heart, Father, help me continually to seek You before Your benefits, to pray for others even before myself, to ask for more power rather than for less pain. And may Your name be glorified now and always.   Amen.

ELEVENTH HEALING SERVICE

The Lord's Prayer

The Bible Reading

"They now brought Him a man whom a demon had made blind and dumb. He cured him and the dumb man spoke and saw. All the people were astounded. 'Can this be David's son?' they asked. But when the Pharisees heard, they said, 'If the man casts demons out, it's only through Beelzebub their prince'.

But Jesus, who knew what they were thinking, said to them: 'If I cast out demons through Beelzebub, through whom do your own people cast them out? You stand condemned by *them*. On the other hand, if I cast out demons through the Spirit of God, it would seem that the Kingdom of God confronts you' " (Matthew 12).

The Meditation

Christ's contemporaries obviously believed that illness was caused by demons—evil spirits which filled the atmosphere. In some ways this is quite a "convenient" belief, since it seems to relieve man of the responsibility of being well. Today we don't use the word demon, but don't we regard a germ in much the same way? Do *I* not tend to put the blame on germs rather than on my own imprudence or ignorance, forgetting that a large proportion of illnesses are caused from within? As has been said: "Germs are only accessories after the fact", i.e. they derive their power to hurt us from *our* weakness. Isn't it when we're below par that we catch a cold so easily?

It has been claimed that this blind and dumb man was afflicted with a purely emotional form of these ailments. Would this, even if true, reduce the wonder of Christ's power? Not at all. Plainly, the doctors and the religious men of the time were powerless to do anything, which is one reason they tried to minimise the cure when Jesus performed it. They claimed Christ was casting out evil by evil—a rather stupid argument which Christ was quick to point out to them.

No, Christ's power, so unmistakenly demonstrated here, is the power of Good—the power which is eternally directed against evil in all its forms, including sickness. Demons exist only to be cast out; sickness exists only to be healed. "If I cast out demons through the Spirit of God," Jesus says, "it would seem that the Kingdom of God confronts you."

How true that is! Wherever His Spirit is at work, God's Kingdom is there. It's here in my generation. It's here in my heart, for has He not cast out the demons of resentment and fear, even if not the demons of disease and pain? And this is just the first fruits of His power working within me. For He has promised to overcome evil with good. But it's for me to help Him this far: not just to believe that He can cure my infirmity, but to believe that He will.

My Prayer for Today

O Light of men, I confess my blindness to the full glory of Your power, and pray You to open the eyes of my understanding to acknowledge You as the Son of God with power. O Word of God, I confess that I have stood dumb before the clear revelation of Your love towards me, as declared in the Gospel, and pray You to open my mouth that I might show forth Your praise.

Bless the doctors and surgeons of our land, and help me to have greater confidence in mine.

Bless the scientists and chemists of our land, and help me to be grateful for any healing agency they may discover.

Bless all preachers and other witnesses to the Faith, and help me to know and to feel the power they seek to proclaim.

Hear me, Father, as I pray for those who suffer from the great affliction of blindness. Grant that as they pray for light for the body, they may give thanks for the light of the soul. Bless those who suffer from the great affliction of dumbness. Grant that as they pray for the opening of their mouths, they may give thanks for the opening of their hearts.

Be with the pained in body, and those who are sick in mind. Be with those who have convinced themselves there is no betterment for them, and with those who have foolishly come to believe in their sickness as a punishment sent from You. And be with those of my personal friends who know neither wholeness of body nor of soul, and grant that the love of these my prayers may be taken up into Your great love and used for their healing. (*Silent prayer*)

Amen.

TWELFTH HEALING SERVICE

The Lord's Prayer
The Bible Reading

"Now there came a man called Jairus, a governor of the synagogue, who threw himself down at Jesus' feet and begged him to come to his house because he had an only daughter about twelve years of age, who was dying. Then someone from the synagogue official's house came up and said: 'Your daughter is dead. Don't trouble the Master'. But Jesus heard and said to Jairus: 'Don't be afraid. Only have faith and she shall be saved'.

When He reached the house He allowed no one to go in with Him but Peter, John, and James, and the father and mother of the girl. They were all wailing and beating their breast for her. But He said: 'Wail no more. She is not dead, but asleep'. They laughed at Him, knowing that she was dead. But he seized her hand and cried: 'Little girl, get up!' Her spirit returned, she rose immediately, and He ordered her some food" (Luke 8).

The Meditation

Many people try to explain this story by

denying that the child was really dead. But everyone in the story, including Jesus, knew she was dead; and Christ's comment "she isn't dead but only asleep" cannot be taken to contradict this, since He meant simply that the little girl's death wasn't irrevocable. If we humans can sometimes bring a person back to life by artificial respiration, as happens in cases of drowning, is it reasonable to doubt Christ's power to infuse life again into an inert body?

Yet, like Jairus, *I* have been afraid and have lacked faith. Whether actually near to death or not, I have laughed at the very prospect of finding relief from my particular complaint. But even supposing I *do* die. What then? Is that the end? "No," cries St. Paul, "for the trumpet shall sound and the dead shall be raised incorruptible, and we shall all be changed . . . for this mortal must put on immortality."

Now I know in my heart that those who have this kind of faith actually have the best chance of recovery in *this* life. I know that by leaving my sickness in His hands, there's a far better chance of finding new strength than if I despair and become resentful. But can I make this act of faith? Indeed I can! For is not God the God of love? And is not Christ the Lord of life?

My Prayer for Today

I pray You, Lord, to teach me to listen more carefully to the Voice which whispers in my ear

"Do not be afraid, only have faith"—and help me to recognise its authority. Inspire me to remember those times past when You called me back to life from the grave beneath, and may this recognition of past mercies help me to lay hold more firmly upon Your great promises for the future.

In all my suffering and pain, Gracious Father, give me the prayerful support of my friends; casting out from them, as well as from me, that attitude which restricts the flow of Your healing waters. And grant that I may never become so self-centred as to forget to pray for others who suffer as much as, or even more than, I do.

> You love us at all times, Father; yet, if we love others, Your love to us is bound to be more real.

> You desire to heal us, Father; yet, if we fervently desire the healing of others, our spirits will better tune in to Yours.

> You hold out the offer of forgiveness, Father; yet, if we're always ready to forgive others, we'll know better the power of that forgiveness.

Grant now, O God, that I may cast fewer shadows across Your light—the shadows of unbelief and fearfulness and despair. Grant now that I may put fewer barriers in the way of Your love—the barriers of resentment and peevishness and self-concern. And grant me to know that nothing—neither death nor life—can separate me from You, my Lord and my God.

Amen.

THIRTEENTH HEALING SERVICE

The Lord's Prayer
The Bible Reading

"There was a woman who for twelve years had suffered from a haemorrhage. She had undergone much at the hands of many physicians and had spent all her resources to no good purpose. In fact, she had gone from bad to worse. Now, having heard the stories about Jesus, she came up from behind through the crowd and touched His cloak, for she had been thinking: 'If I can only touch His clothes, I shall be saved'. On the instant, her haemorrhage was staunched and she could feel that she was cured of the affliction.

She came and fell at His feet and told Him the whole truth. Whereupon He said: 'Daughter, your faith has saved you. Go now in peace, and be rid of your affliction' " (Mark 5).

The Meditation

Is there a flavour of magic in this vivid picture of an instantaneous healing? Emphatically not! The woman wasn't healed by the clothes, but by the Wearer, through confidence in Him.

Yet there's always a danger of adopting this magical attitude to healing. Was it a mature Christian faith that this woman had, or was it merely a case of suggestion? Whatever our answer may be, the crucial fact is that it was the Lord's doing and "marvellous in our eyes".

Perhaps a disciple had told her of Jesus, and this would understandably awaken expectations in the woman's heart. Most people's faith has come as a result of hearing God's word preached or witnessed to. That is surely true of myself — and certainly I have great expectations of Jesus!

Now, however much I may have undergone at the hands of the medical profession, I am well aware I mustn't regard this story as a slight upon that profession. Maybe without my doctor I'd be a lot worse! And if I had more confidence in him, maybe I'd be a great deal better. In any event I must try now to bring Christ not the remains of my faith but a faith in full flower; not the spent fragments of my vigour and my hope, but the full power of my spirit.

This woman was cured on the instant; but I haven't succumbed to the temptation to expect Him to heal by the same pattern every time. It's my privilege to pray in faith for healing; it's His privilege to heal in the way He thinks best. And I believe He will do so.

My Prayer for Today

O You who are the Great Physician of my

body, and the Wonderful Saviour of my soul, forbid that any trial of body or soul might make me less confident of Your mercy and less sure of Your love. Hold the vision of wholeness and peace before me; and, when I have attained to it, make my heart sing with praise and with joy, for Your name's sake.

O God of compassion, bless those of my fellow-sufferers who have undergone much at the hands of many physicians, and seem to feel no betterment. Keep them from resentment — as You have kept me. Keep them from despair — as You have kept me. Keep them from cynicism — as You have kept me. And as my love goes out to them in prayer, may Your love come into me.

For those who are praying for me, and for fellow-sufferers, I pray, O God; for all healers who, in different ways, are ministers of Your redeeming power; for those who preach the Word of Forgiveness, that this Word might be received in faith, and be a refreshment to the body as well as to the soul. And I pray for those who seek You only as a last resort, that, in finding a cure for their bodies, they may also find a resting-place for their souls. For Jesus' sake.

Amen.

FOURTEENTH HEALING SERVICE

The Lord's Prayer

The Bible Reading

"They went into Capernaum and on the first Sabbath He entered the synagogue and taught. His way of teaching filled them with amazement, for He taught them like one with authority, and not like the doctors of the Law.

That very day, in their synagogue, there was a man possessed by an unclean spirit who cried out: 'What is Your business with us, Jesus the Nazarene? Have You come to destroy us? We know who You are, the Holy One of God.' Jesus rounded on him. 'Hold your tongue', He said, 'and come out of the man.' The unclean spirit convulsed the man, gave a loud cry, and came out of him.

All were amazed. 'What have we here?' they said, as they talked the matter over. 'A new doctrine this, and it has power behind it. He even tells unclean spirits what to do, and they obey Him' " (Mark 1).

The Meditation

I wonder if *I* have kept my sense of

amazement at His way of teaching? or have I become so familiar with the facts of the Faith that the unique Figure of the Teacher Himself has become just a little hazy in my eyes? One thing is sure: by losing my amazement at the uniqueness of His teachings in the Scriptures, I shall automatically blind myself to the vision of Him as the Great Physician.

The men present in the synagogue weren't slow to see the connection between Christ's preaching and His healing power. It wasn't just a spoken word, but an acted word as well. Yet many people today are slow to see the connection between accepting the truths of the Gospel and accepting His gift of healing. They cannot quite realise just how saving a belief it is that God loves them to the uttermost, or that He's willing to forgive the blackest sin. And yet the benefits of such beliefs for *physical* health are too well authenticated to be doubted any longer. Yet, maybe *I* still doubt?

Whatever else the story of the possessed man at Capernaum means, it certainly brings the stimulating reminder that my unclean spirit must give way to the holy power of Christ. This man, of course, was in a highly abnormal psychological state; and yet isn't it true that the bad in *every* man is able to recognise perfect Goodness? And isn't it true that *every* man has some sin or other which he is reluctant for Christ to destroy?

Mustn't I hope today that this reluctance isn't preventing my physical healing, far less my spiritual healing? And may I not hope, on the other hand, that by my daily worship and reading of the Scriptures, the Figure of Christ may at last present itself to me in such holiness and power that my unclean spirit may be rebuked as finally and as wonderfully as that of the possessed man of Capernaum? Can I doubt that this is what He longs to do for me — if I'll give Him what cooperation I'm able?

My Prayer for Today

O You who alone can create a clean heart and renew a right spirit within me, I come to You today for cleansing and renewal. I have been possessed by the spirit of fear, and crave now the spirit of faith. I have been possessed by the spirit of heaviness, and I crave now the spirit of buoyancy. I have been possessed by the spirit of resentment, and crave now the spirit of Love.

There's nothing I can give You, Father, in thankfulness for Your care of me, except myself. Help me to give that. May I see that You desire no return for Your love, except to watch me living a life of love. Grant me now and always to leave the issues of each day trustfully in Your hands, believing implicitly in Your will to heal me.

O Lord of All Being, save me from being possessed by the spirit of pride and self-reliance.

O Creator of Beauty, save me from being possessed by the spirit of impurity and imperfection.

O Author of Blessing, save me from being possessed by the spirit of apathy and ingratitude.

Hear me, Father, as I commend to You those who suffer from malignant disease (*silent prayer*); those who suffer from split-personality or other mental affliction (*silent prayer*); those who suffer from what they regard as an incurable disease (*silent prayer*). May they be raised to a new vision and a new hope; and may they know the difference between resigning themselves to their sickness and resigning themselves to You. Amen.

FIFTEENTH HEALING SERVICE

The Lord's Prayer

The Bible Reading

"On another Sabbath day when He went to the synagogue and taught, there was a man whose right hand was withered, and the doctors and Pharisees watched Him closely to see whether He would heal on the Sabbath, hoping to have a charge to bring against Him. But He knew their thoughts and said to the man with the withered hand: 'Rise, and stand here in the centre'.

The man rose and stood there, and Jesus said to them: 'I put a question to you. Are we permitted on the Sabbath to choose between doing good and doing evil, saving a life and destroying it?' Then, after looking at each of them in turn, He said to the man: 'Hold out your hand'. He did so, and his hand was made sound once more" (Luke 6).

The Meditation

The question which many sufferers asked at the time of Christ's ministry on earth was whether it was right for them to be healed at all, far less on the Sabbath. How tragic that there should be any doubt about God's willingness to heal at *any* time! I know He wants to heal my affliction — but maybe I doubt His ability. If so, it's worth looking at this simple but vivid story of an instantaneous cure.

I see at once that the man himself played quite a large part in his cure. Jesus could easily have come over to him and performed the healing without asking him to rise to his feet. But He didn't. He asked him first of all to "rise and stand here in the centre". Perhaps that's the request He makes to me? And perhaps I've wanted Him to come over and heal me as I sat at ease? Certainly I've tried to keep praying, but I have been greatly tempted to want a healing at minimum inconvenience to myself.

I'm impressed, moreover, by the fact that it never occurred to Jesus that the man wouldn't respond positively to His suggestions. Yes, Jesus had faith in the man, just as the man had faith in Him. This is one of the most important factors in non-physical healing, and one that's often forgotten or minimised. Can I be totally unconcerned that Jesus has faith in me?

But, granted my faith in Him, can I expect that I'll be "made sound once more"? Maybe not immediately. Maybe there's a whole work of repair to be done first. Maybe a slow cure is God's way of ensuring my continual growth in grace. But His will is to heal, and His work is to heal — so what hinders me from being healed?

My Prayer for Today

O You who give yourself to me, help me daily to give myself to You.

O You who believe in me, help me daily to believe in You as Saviour.

O You who seek to possess me, help me daily to seek to be possessed.

Gracious Father, You bid me pray in Christ's name. Grant then that I may pray, having cast out all undue self-concern. Grant that I may never pray in the hope of simply making use of You, but that I may be made use of by You. And grant that I may think, say, and do only those things of which You would approve.

You, Heavenly King, are the vanquisher of sin. Conquer it in me.

You, Heavenly Sympathiser, are the dispeller of sorrow. Lift it away from me.

You, Heavenly Healer, are the rescuer from sickness. Perform this for me.

But lest my prayer should not avail because of selfishness, hear me as I pray for those sharing the fellowship of suffering; and let this prayer arise not because I believe it will help me only, but because I feel the privilege of speaking with You, my Father, about those who do so deeply concern me. Bless each one, I pray. And bless those who tend them; for Jesus' sake.   Amen.

SIXTEENTH HEALING SERVICE

The Lord's Prayer

The Bible Reading

"On the journey to Jerusalem He passed between Samaria and Galilee, and as He came to one of the villages, He was faced by ten lepers, who kept their distance and called across to Him: 'Jesus, Master! have pity on us'. Directly He saw them He said: 'Go and show yourselves to the priests', with the result that, as they went, they were cleansed.

And one of them, seeing that he was cured, turned back with a great cry of praise to God, prostrated Himself at Jesus' feet and thanked Him. This man was a Samaritan. Jesus asked: 'Were not all ten cleansed? Where are the other nine? Can it be true that none of them except this foreigner has come back to give glory to God?' And to the man He said: 'Rise and go. Your faith has saved you' " (Luke 17).

The Meditation

I can't read this story without linking it with the story of the *one* leper whom Jesus healed immediately—and the difference in the time factor is suggestive. For here the lepers are cleansed "as they went", i.e. by a different method than that employed in the case of the one leper, and yet by the same power. Here we have a firm refutation of the idea that the same healing technique can be applied to each and every illness, as some "faith-healers" claim.

Christ may heal me in a different way from my fellow-sufferer — which is worth remembering. Certainly I must know of someone who was "cleansed as he went", perhaps coming for a "laying on of hands" or coming to worship, as I'm now doing, and although nothing happened immediately, by the time he had got home his ailment was greatly relieved or gone altogether. But perhaps there's also a mild rebuke for me in this story. For, haven't I been tempted to think I should be cleansed *as I lay* and not *as I went*, and that Christ should heal without any help from me? Often He does heal without help from people, but am I right in *expecting* Him to do it in that way for me? Christ wants as much faith and love from me as He can get, for even the power of God sometimes works more smoothly with the oil of man's faith.

One thing is sure: I cannot be really whole — saved in body, mind, and soul — without the profound faith of this thankful Samaritan. Bodily healing *may* come without faith, but not the salvation of my soul. These nine healed men were healed only in one sense, but the

Samaritan was healed in every sense! The question which remains for me, then, is this: Is my aim the healing of my body or the healing of my whole being?

My Prayer for Today

Hear my prayer, Father, as I lay before You the faith which believes that You exist, and grant me also that faith which believes that You can heal. I know that sickness doesn't come from You, but give me also to know that it can actually arise through the *absence* of Yourself! I believe, Father, that You will heal me; yet, if healing doesn't come, let me still believe in You.

- O Dispeller of men's fears, graciously take away my fear of the unknown, that I may rest confidently in Your loving purpose for me.
- O Destroyer of men's fantasies, graciously rebuke me for my wrong ideas of You, that I may know You as You are.
- O Deliverer of men's frailties, graciously send the healing power of Your Spirit into me, that I may give you the glory.

For all the work of healing which constantly and lovingly is prosecuted in this world of Yours, I pray today. May those who suffer or feel at the end of their strength feel the power of the Lord. Bless those who, even today, may turn to You as Saviour and find peace of soul. (*Silent prayer*)

Now grant, Lord, that my thoughts may be pure, my words clean, and my deeds noble, so that even as I witness quietly for You here, Your will may be done in me. Keep my heart ever open to the warmth of Your love. Keep my mind ever open to the power of Your truth. And keep my will ever ready to be changed by Yours. Through Jesus Christ, my healing Saviour.

Amen.

SEVENTEENTH HEALING SERVICE

The Lord's Prayer

The Bible Reading

"A centurion there had a slave who was sick—indeed, he was at death's door. His master set great store by him, and so, having heard about Jesus, he sent Him a deputation of Jewish elders begging Him to come and save his servant. These presented themselves to Jesus and earnestly besought Him. They said: 'The man is one who has deserved this kindness at your hands, for he loves our people and he built us our synagogue himself.'

Jesus went with them and had nearly reached the house when the centurion sent Him a message by some friends. 'Lord,' he said, 'do not put yourself out. I'm not worthy to receive you under my roof. Nor, for that reason, did I presume to come to you myself; but you have only to say the word and my boy will be cured.'

When He heard this, Jesus was amazed at the man; and turning to the crowd that followed Him, He said: 'I tell you, not even in Israel have I found such faith'. And the messengers, when they got back to the house, found the slave in perfect health" (Luke 7).

The Meditation

Here surely is a vivid illustration of a wonderful fact that has become increasingly apparent to some prayer groups—"absent healing". To God, distance is no object. Science may be sceptical of the very possibility, but any who hold this view surely have a faulty conception of God. Wasn't I told in childhood that God is everywhere? God's healing waves don't have to come from a local transmitter set up in a particular place in heaven! They're there all the time. As the hymn says: 'God is always near me'. And it's my responsibility to do all I can to remove the barriers which are keeping Him and His curative rays from penetrating into my body—and into my soul.

To return to the Gospel story, there's one lovely touch worth noting. Even the Jews pleaded for the Gentile. And can I doubt that these solicitings were far from superfluous? Can I doubt, indeed, that the love of the centurion for the slave was an important factor in Christ's willingness to come to heal him? In God's providence, man's love for his fellow has a curative property. Aren't there those who love me and are praying for me now with all the fervour of that love? In face of that fact, mustn't my own faith be stirred up to greater warmth and effectiveness? Yes, my lukewarmness, my reluctance to believe in the power of prayer, may be nullifying their work on my behalf. But I'll see that this doesn't happen now!

My Prayer for Today

O Source of healing power, I gladly turn to You for strength of heart.

O Source of liberating joy, I gladly turn to You for buoyancy of spirit.

O Source of deep composure, I gladly turn to You for serenity of mind.

Grant, O Father, that I might be surrounded by the love not just of heaven, but also of earth; that I might know it to be not only Your will for me to be healed, but also the will of my friends. May I be as confident of Your love as You are of my cure. May I seek Your help as earnestly as You desire to give it. May I give myself to You as unreservedly as You give Yourself to me.

And since all sufferers are bound together in a sacred fellowship, I would pray for my fellow-sufferers today, asking that the same power which is mightily at work in me this minute might be manifest in them to dispel the shadows of life. (*Silent prayer*) I pray for Your blessing on the gracious work of healing in all places—and to Your name may all the glory be given, now and always.   Amen.

EIGHTEENTH HEALING SERVICE

The Lord's Prayer

The Bible Reading

"As He left the town (Jericho) with His disciples and a large following, there was a blind beggar, Bartimaeus, sitting by the road. Learning that this was Jesus the Nazarene, he began to cry out: 'Son of David, Jesus, have pity on me'. A number of people told him to hold his tongue, but this only made him cry out the more. 'Son of David, have pity on me!'

Jesus stopped and said: 'Call him'. So they called the blind man. 'All is well,' they said to him. 'Get up; He is calling you.' Bartimaeus threw off his cloak, leapt to his feet and came to Jesus. Jesus said to him: 'What do you wish me to do for you?' 'To make me see again, Rabboni', said the blind man. 'Go now,' said Jesus, 'your faith has saved you.' His sight came back at once and he followed Him along the road" (Mark 10).

The Meditation

How wonderful it is to be able to see and understand the printed page! Perhaps it's a story like this which reminds me how often my prayers of asking crowd out the prayers of thanks that should accompany them. Could it be that I've been spending all my time praying for myself, when half my time praying for others might have brought more positive results? Could it be that a genuine prayer of thanksgiving for the gift of sight—or for any other faculty that I have *not* lost—might do me more good than an exaggerated self-concern? This is worth a thought.

But whatever my trouble is, this story brings me more than a grain of comfort; for Christ is neither blind to my need, nor deaf to my call. The power that restored a blind man's sight is the same power which can drive out the pains of *my* flesh. Do I really want that power to work in me, so that God's glory may be manifest? Then perhaps I should be encouraged by the reward of perseverance given to blind Bartimaeus. "Son of David, have pity on me!" And Christ did have pity. Shouldn't I rejoice that, in God's providence, a person's faith can help to heal him?

This story is the last healing miracle recorded in St. Mark's Gospel. But miracles aren't confined to New Testament times. They happen now. They even happen to people like me. "Go now," says Jesus, "your faith has saved you".

My Prayer for Today

Merciful Father, today won't be without its mercies, and not the least of them will be the fact that others are praying for me. Hear me now as I pray for them. There are many mercies to which I have been blind. Hear me, then, as I confess that insensitiveness to Your love for which not even my ailment is sufficient excuse; my readiness to listen to those who say that there's no help for him in God; the tendency to self-pity which aggravates my complaint and blinds me even more to Your love.

Spirit of Light, dispel my darkness.

Spirit of Love, dispel my fears.

Spirit of Life, dispel my unresponsiveness.

Move within me now, O healing power. Bring strength where there was weakness. Bring betterment where there was worsening. Bring wholeness where there was incompleteness. Teach me how to yield myself unreservedly to You. Give me the feeling of utter dependence upon You. Nourish in me the hope and the expectancy which You Yourself graciously use to heal. Preserve me from setting a time-limit for You, or from thinking that a cure is highly unlikely. And let nothing disturb my faith in the power of prayer—or in You.   Amen.

NINETEENTH HEALING SERVICE

The Lord's Prayer

The Bible Reading

"On a Sabbath day, when He had gone into the house of one of the leading Pharisees for a meal, and they were watching Him closely, a man who suffered from dropsy appeared before Him. Whereupon Jesus said to the lawyers and Pharisees: 'Is it lawful to heal on the Sabbath or not?' They were silent; and He laid hold of him, cured him, and dismissed him.

Then He said to them: 'Which of *you* on the Sabbath, when his donkey or ox falls into a well, will not immediately pull him out?' To which they were unable to reply" (Luke 14).

The Meditation

How strange it seems to anyone living today that there could be any question of God not condoning the healing of a sick man on the grounds that it was the Sabbath! This surely is religion run riot. Yet many people make another mistake which is hardly less excusable: namely, believing that there are some diseases which God doesn't wish to cure on *any* day. The

Jews did at least believe that it was right to heal on weekdays, whereas some people actually believe God has sent them a particular illness or infirmity which He has no intention they should be rid of! This too is religion run riot.

Jesus made it crystal clear that sickness is always to be fought as something evil. But, alas, some people may be denying themselves healing simply because they have convinced themselves that God doesn't will to heal them. But He does! The blockage is not at God's end, but at theirs.

Maybe it was just a functional complaint that this man had. But was it any less the power of Christ that healed him? Mustn't I, in any case, believe that if I allow Christ to "lay hold of me", He will "cure me and dismiss me"? In face of the overwhelming evidence of New Testament cures and of those achieved in modern times, how can I hold back? For Jesus saves! Not just soul, but body too. Not just from an unhealthy conscience, but from an unhealthy mind or body as well.

My Prayer for Today

There are many things, Father, that I have to confess today: my tendency to forget Your love for me; my hesitancy to believe in Your will for me to be healed; my aptitude for over-anxiety or for a too ready submission to what I mistakenly call my fate. I confess my reluctance to accept the forgiveness I badly need, my refusal to believe in the power of my friends' prayers on my behalf, my inability to turn away from self—and I'm sorry for these faults, O Saviour Christ.

But now, having accepted Your pardon, may I find Your peace. Having felt Your love, may I see Your light. Having acknowledged Your favour to me, may I know Your faithfulness to do that which You have promised. Help me now to pray for those known to me who are in pain or distress today, and minister to their needs. (*Silent prayer*) And help me, Lord, to remember that there are some who are praying for me, and that You hear their prayers.

Preserve me, O God, from the sin of wanting healing more than You; from the folly of thinking my daily worship is a short cut to health; from the presumption of testing You by the measure of success or failure which attends my devotions. For I praise You, Lord Jesus, for what You are before I praise You for what You do!

Accept my praise now, I pray, and of Your mercy use it as a channel of renewal and redemption. In the coming days help me to co-operate in the fullest confidence with those who seek my health through medical channels, knowing that all true healing is of You. Through Jesus Christ my Lord.   Amen.

TWENTIETH HEALING SERVICE

The Lord's Prayer

The Bible Reading

"He went to His own part of the country, accompanied by His disciples. When the Sabbath came round He began to teach in the synagogue, and most of them when they heard Him were confounded. They said: 'Where did the man get this from? What is this wisdom that has been given Him, and these miracles that are brought about through Him?' But Jesus said to them: 'A prophet is not without honour except in his own country, his own family, and his own house'. And He was unable to do there any miracle of note, though He did lay hands on a few sick people and cure them. He was amazed at their lack of faith.

Then He summoned the Twelve to Him and began to send them out in pairs on missions, giving them authority over unclean spirits. So they set forth and preached, to bring men to repentance, and from time to time cast many demons out and anointed many sick with oil and cured them" (Mark 6).

The Meditation

It's one of the sadder features of life that familiarity so often breeds incredulity, if not contempt. Maybe *I* have become so familiar with Christ that, in spite of myself, I have become "inoculated" against the infection of faith. I know Him as Friend, and in so doing I may have blinded myself to His Kingship. I know Him as Saviour of my soul, and in so doing I may have pushed into the background the fact that He is also the Healer of my body.

These men who tried to soft-pedal Christ's achievements were clearly guilty of deliberate blindness. They *ought* not to have marvelled so much, for they knew the reports that had been coming in about His previous mighty works. They *ought* not to have tried to throw cold water on His achievements, for His upbringing simply had nothing to do with the point at issue, namely, was He or was He not capable of doing the things that were reported of Him?

Yet, haven't *I* some preconceived notions about what He can and cannot do? Perhaps I believe He can heal functional disorders but not organic ones? Perhaps I believe He can heal by laying on of hands but not through prayer alone? Certainly I must at least consider whether Christ is unable to heal me because of my halfhearted faith. The question for me seems to be: Is He amazed at *my* lack of faith? If so, maybe it's because I recognise Him as only a prophet, and not the Saviour. "Lord, I believe; help my unbelief!"

My Prayer for Today

Lord Jesus Christ, You who sent out Your disciples to bring people to repentance, hear my confession and restore to me the joy of Your salvation. If I have developed a partial immunity to the great love which You have towards me, bring upon me the infection of a fervent spirit, that I may know You as Saviour and serve You as Lord. If I have been deceiving myself with the belief that I needed no forgiveness, but only healing, reveal to me my deepest need and help me to see that You can meet it.

Hear me, Lord, as I pray for those whom You have sent out in this generation with authority over unclean spirits—that their word may have healing in its wings; for it's Your word. May their ministrations bring health and happiness, for this is Your purpose of love for all people. Be with all doctors and nurses and psychiatrists, and with those who heal through their love and their prayers. Give skill to their hands, wisdom to their minds, gentleness to their hearts; and give them a sense of privilege in being co-workers with You.

Hear me, Father, as I pray in the silence of my heart for those known to me—and those unknown—who lie in pain or grief. (*Silent prayer*) Bless them, and bless me, O Saviour Christ.

Amen.

TWENTY-FIRST
HEALING SERVICE

The Lord's Prayer
The Bible Reading

"On leaving the synagogue He went into
Simon's house. Now Simon's mother-in-law was
suffering from high fever and they consulted
Him about her. Jesus, standing over her,
rebuked the fever and it left her. She got up
immediately and began to wait on them. As the
sun set, all those with friends who were suffering
from this or that disease brought them to Him;
and He cured them, laying His hands on every
one" (Luke 4).

The Meditation

It's strange how many people in serious
distress consult everyone except the Lord of Life
Himself! So often He's a last resort. Sometimes,
no doubt, people fail to consult Christ because
they don't want to "bother" Him; and yet this
betrays the very thing that's lacking—a belief in
a personal Christ, a belief in a Christ who cares
to the extent of *not* being bothered by any
request prompted by genuine need.

How natural and how right that they "consulted Him about her". And how natural that "He rebuked the fever and it left her". How was it done? We don't know. What exactly was the fever? We don't know. But we do know that, whereas no one else was able to help Simon's mother-in-law, Christ was. It has of course been claimed by some people that hypnotic suggestion can check fevers, but however we try to explain this cure — or explain it away — nothing can take away from its wonder as a demonstration of divine power.

And it's the same Saviour that I'm called on to love and believe in now — the Saviour who "heals all my diseases, who redeems my life from destruction". Perhaps He will do it by a word, if He deems it appropriate. Perhaps He will cure me through a devout healer, by the laying on of hands. Or He may heal me through the fervent prayers of those who love me. Whichever way He chooses, one thing He desires in me: the fervency of faith which is prepared to believe in Him whether or not He heals. Do I have this kind of faith?

My Prayer for Today

O Comforter of men, my Father, I come into Your presence with a heart made joyful by the remembrance of Your great goodness to me. Even in the midst of discomfort and pain, I have found Your peace. Even amid perplexity

120

and anguish of soul, I have felt Your healing touch.

Yet, I haven't always lived on the summit of faith. There are times when I have doubted, and I've heard Your whispered rebuke. There are times when I have been afraid, and You have reminded me of the perfect love which casts out fear. There are times when I have been loveless and full of self-concern, and I could have wept for shame. Of Your mercy, not only forgive me, Lord, but renew a right spirit within me.

O You who are King of Glory, manifest Your power in me!

O You who are Creator of Goodness, fill me with all good!

O You who are Bringer of Gladness, make me to rejoice in You!

Hear me, Father, as I pray for others too. For I am bound with all sufferers in the holy fellowship of suffering, and know it's Your will for our prayers to help one another. Support those who are unable to walk. Rebuke the fevers and diseases which lay us so low. Give peace to those who suffer from nervous and mental troubles. And bless those whom I remember in the silence of my heart now. (*Silent prayer*)

Amen.

TWENTY-SECOND
HEALING SERVICE

The Lord's Prayer

The Bible Reading

"Leaving the district of Tyre, He returned by way of Sidon to the Sea of Galilee across the territory of the Ten Towns. They brought Him a deaf man who could hardly speak, and begged Him to lay His hand on him. He took the man away from the crowd by himself, thrust His fingers into his ears, spat, and touched his tongue. Then, looking up into the heavens, He gave a sigh and said to the man *Ephphatha*, which means 'be opened'.

The man's ears were opened, and the impediment to his speech was removed, and he spoke clearly. Jesus commanded them to tell no one, but the more He did so, the more eagerly they published the news. In fact, they were astonished beyond measure. They said: 'How perfectly He has done everything! He not only makes deaf people hear, but He makes dumb people talk!' " (Mark 7)

The Meditation

Here's a story rich with suggestion. Many

people today regard deafness and dumbness as among the ailments considered to come into the category of incurable, and it seems clear that Christ's contemporaries thought so. Yet today there are many instances of the healing of the deaf and dumb by non-physical means.

However, this story isn't recorded only for the benefit of the deaf and dumb. It was written down by St. Mark in order to "carry the mind along to that larger ministry of making mind and heart more sensitive to the voice of God". This is a ministry that we all need, whatever our special ailment might be. Indeed, isn't it even possible that my physical ailment has been aggravated by my spiritual deafness to the still small voice of God?

Whether or not this is so, I certainly should remember the promise that both the physical ears and the spiritual ears of the deaf shall be unstopped! I note that in this story Jesus was careful to take His patient out of the reach of those who might deride the very idea of a cure; and perhaps in my case He would love to "take me aside" and in the quietness of my room work His miracle of love. But he doesn't want me to be one of "God's mutes". He wants me to rejoice in His love for me and to *believe* He can heal me.

I see from this story that Christ didn't heal with a word. I see also that He didn't scorn to use what psychologists would call "suggestion".

Maybe that is to be His way with me? Maybe He knows that to heal me gradually will be most beneficial for my total spiritual experience. Maybe He even knows that, by responding to His suggestion, I can play a substantial part in the cure He has ready for me. Certainly it's to me too, right now, that He's saying "Be opened"—not just my ears and mouth, but my heart and mind!

My Prayer for Today

Hear me, merciful Saviour, as I confess my deafness to Your promise of deliverance; as I confess how often I have stood dumb in face of some token of Your saving goodness. Forgive me if I have got used to the idea of being unwell. Forgive me if I have thought to *deserve* a speedy cure. Forgive me if I have failed to respond to the treatment in which You would have me share. Help me now to give myself more wholeheartedly to Your wisdom, in the knowledge that You do everything well.

My prayers for fellow-sufferers are so often weak and unreal, O God! Fill them now with passion and concern, that in the outgoing of my spirit, healing may come not just to others, but to myself.

You fill all things, Creator Spirit; fill me with Life.

You care for all things, Father God; fill me with Love.

You illumine all things, Sun of my soul; fill me with Light.

Grant me today and every day to seek Your Kingdom above all things—and I shall find that wholeness will be added to me. Help me to understand more fully Your purpose of love for all men, and grant that where I am tempted to doubt, You will confirm my faith; that where I am tempted to despair, You will raise my hopes; that where I am tempted to complain to You, You will give me the grace of patience and courage. And now to You, the power of my life, be all honour and glory, now and always.

Amen.

TWENTY-THIRD
HEALING SERVICE

The Lord's Prayer

The Bible Reading

"When they came down from the mountains, He was met by a large crowd; and out of the gathering came a man's voice. 'Master,' he cried, 'I beg you to look at my son who is the only one I have. A spirit seizes him and gives a sudden cry; it rends him till he foams at the mouth; and as the convulsions slowly subside, it leaves him shattered. I begged your disciples to cast it out, but they couldn't.'

At this Jesus exclaimed: 'O faithless and perverse generation! How much longer must I be with you and bear with you? Bring your son here.' The lad was still on his way to Jesus when the demon flung him down and convulsed him. But Jesus rebuked the unclean spirit and cured the lad; then gave him back to his father. And all were filled with awe at the majesty of God" (Luke 9).

The Meditation

How natural that a father should forget the hundreds around him and beg for his epileptic son! No self-consciousness, no hesitancy, no feeling of doing something wrong in stealing the limelight, as it were. This is a picture which brings me a reminder — a reminder that I must never delay in asking help for myself or a loved one on the grounds that Jesus has plenty on His mind without *my* trouble. Christ is the God of the individual.

Mustn't I be quite sure that it's not only God's command that I bring my deepest needs before Him, but also His promise that they will be met? Far from my not troubling Him being a sign of deeper piety, it's actually a proof that I don't know God as Father at all!

Wasn't it because this man stood in the right relationship with Jesus that He was willing to perform this marvellous cure? The father's faith helped to create the right "atmosphere" or context for the healing; and it was because the disciples didn't have this faith that they received this rather stern rebuke. Maybe *my* faith is insufficient to create this atmosphere?

Whether or not this was a case of epilepsy as we know it today, the story makes very plain that it took nothing less than Christ's healing power to cure it. The bystanders were rightly "filled with awe at the majesty of God". Shouldn't *I* be similarly filled with awe at the mere reading of this wonderful story? For, it's intended to be a pointer to *my* cure, and to evoke my faith in that cure. Has it done so?

My Prayer for Today

You desire me, O God, to bring a mature faith to You; yet preserve me from the error of holding back just because I haven't got it. You desire me to wish and to pray for wholeness of soul as well as of body; yet preserve me from an exaggerated sense of shame when I can only summon the strength to ask for the latter. You desire me to love You for Yourself more than for what You can give me; yet preserve me from the failure to praise You for Your benefits just because I cannot so far praise You for Yourself.

Grant, O Lord, that even as I worship You in these daily devotions I may find my faith deepened, my love broadened, and my life enriched. Grant that I may not only believe in Christ's healing power at work within me, but may be fully conscious of Him, and may give Him a freer course in my pained body and my restless soul.

Lord Jesus, give me hope for hopelessness!
Lord Jesus, give me love for lovelessness!
Lord Jesus, give me life for lifelessness!

For the healing ministry of Your Church I pray today, O God; that she may not be distracted or disheartened either by her own failures or by her many critics. For doctors and nurses, psychiatrists and psychologists, and for all workers among the sick, I pray; that a sense of vocation may be upon them, and the power of Your Spirit be with them.

Bless those who are sick and cannot offer You the faith which I can; and help me to realise my responsibility for them by offering that faith on their behalf. Bless those who shall suffer agony tonight, and grant them the grace of courage and of undying hope. For Jesus' sake.   Amen.

TWENTY-FOURTH HEALING SERVICE

The Lord's Prayer

The Bible Reading

"As they left Jericho a large crowd followed Him; and there were two blind men sitting by the road, who when they heard that Jesus was passing cried out: 'Lord, have pity on us, Son of David!' People told them to hold their tongues, but this only made them cry out all the louder: 'Lord, have pity on us, Son of David!'

Jesus stopped, called them to Him and said: 'What do you wish me to do for you?' 'Lord,' they said, 'we want our eyes to be opened.' Jesus was moved to compassion and touched their eyes. Their sight came back at once and they followed Him" (Matthew 20).

The Meditation

How typical of Jesus, and how symbolic, that He should turn aside from the large crowd which followed Him to these two needy souls. His whole ministry is full of this wonderful concern and compassion for individuals. I myself may be tempted to think that Christ is more interested in world missions or ecumenical conferences or packed congregations than in my personal distress, but I would be wrong. Christ's question to the two men is His question to me: 'What do you wish me to do for you?' That was his question to blind Bartimaeus—a story so like Matthew's one that it may well be the same incident.

And maybe I should realise that it's not such a superfluous question as it may sound. For, *why* do I want my eyes to be opened? *Why* do I want to be rid of my arthritis or my paralysis or my nervous debility? So that I may again be free to go my own way, or free to give God the greater glory? Significantly enough, the two blind men followed Him after the miracle was performed—which might suggest that their request for sight wasn't a mere request for personal convenience. Don't I myself feel that a cry for help that's coupled with a cry to "help my unbelief" has more chance of availing with God than one prompted by the mere desire for removal of physical pain?

In fact, maybe I'm not physically blind but could be suffering from a far more tragic form of blindness—spiritual blindness. If so, this story can help me to make the right approach. "Lord, have pity on me, Son of David!" And if I do that, I may not only find this spiritual ailment cured at once, but I may also find that half the battle is won for the healing of my physical complaint. One thing is sure: that if I follow Christ *before* I am healed, there's more chance that I will follow Him *after* I'm healed. "Lord, may it be so!"

My Prayer for Today

O You who are sent to heal the broken-hearted, bind up the sorrows of my heart!

O You who are sent to preach deliverance, free me from the tyranny of despair!

O You who are sent to restore men's sight, lighten the darkness of my unbelief!

For those who are seriously ill and going through the valley of the shadow of death, I pray today; for those whose hearts threaten to break with grief; for those who are held captive by infirmity of limb or nerve; for those who are losing all hope of recovery. Give me to know that my prayer on their behalf is not made in vain; and give them to know that they can help themselves through their own prayers. (*Silent prayer*)

You, O God, have worked within me too plainly for me not to acknowledge Your wonderful goodness and Your healing power. You have forgiven me my smallest sin so that I have the peace and joy of a good conscience. You have blessed me with hope when I threatened to despair, with courage when I threatened to submit, with faith when I was becoming afraid—so that I rejoice now in Your fatherly care of me. Grant that every sufferer may share something of this joy, for Christ's sake.

Amen.

TWENTY-FIFTH
HEALING SERVICE

The Lord's Prayer

The Bible Reading

"The next day He arose while it was still dark, and leaving the house made His way into the open country and prayed there for a while. Simon and his companions went in pursuit, found Him, and told Him that everyone was looking for Him. He said to them: 'Let us go elsewhere, to the neighbouring country towns, so that I may preach there also; for that's what I came to do'.

And He went through the whole of Galilee, entering their synagogues to proclaim His message, and casting out demons" (Mark 1).

The Meditation

So often during His ministry Jesus turned aside for periods of prayer, and here is the first recorded occasion when He does so. He had just spent His energies in healing the crowds of sick, and now this expenditure of power has to be followed up by a renewal of power.

If the Healer Himself found this necessary, how much more should I! For I too have spent my energies in enduring my particular cross, in facing up to pain and distress, in trying to sustain the will to live. And unless I do renew my energy in prayer, there may be little alternative to cracking up completely. Prayer isn't an extra; it's the very power of my life.

There's something else which I find suggestive in this passage: Jesus refused to be localised. He refused to become a popular Healer. That surely is the right way to understand His answer to Peter's news that "Everyone was looking for Him". It's intolerable to think that when He said "Let us go elsewhere", He was simply trying to escape from the crowds of sick people who were looking for Him! No, He wanted to extend His preaching and healing ministry as far as He could, to bring the promise of wholeness to as wide a circle as possible. But, just how impressed have *I* been with all this? Have I been inspired with the belief that He is able to cure *me*?

There certainly are some today who think of Jesus as merely a preacher; and yet the record is clear: He "entered their synagogues to proclaim His message" *and* "cast out demons". One thing is sure: however virulent the demon is in my body, Christ has the desire and the power to cast it out. Mustn't I pray and believe that He *will* do this—even for me?

My Prayer for Today

O You who have mastered the art and the secret of prayer, teach me how to pray! So often I have prayed with the mind but not the heart. So often I have prayed and found prayer unreal. So often I have prayed and been rebuked by the selfishness and self-concern of my prayer.

Take my heart, Lord, and let it be consecrated to You.

Take my faith, Lord, and let it be content in You.

Take my frame, Lord, and let it be cured by You.

In all my prayers to You, O God, help me to ask only for those things which would not shame Your purpose, or insult the spiritual image of Yourself which is within me. When I pray for health, may I desire it so that I may enjoy the greater freedom to praise You. When I pray for happiness, may I desire it so that I may share it with others. When I pray for heaven, may I desire it only as the natural fulfilment of that taste of heaven which You have granted me here on earth.

There are many, Father, who need You today. Some hardly know their own needs. Others hardly know You. I pray You to hear my prayer of faith on their behalf now, that they may know strength for weakness, hope for despair, and joy for sorrow. (*Silent prayer*)

Now grant me to know more and more that if I do not have hold of You, I have nothing; and that if You don't have hold of me, I am nothing. And may I live evermore to Your honour and glory. For Jesus' sake.   Amen.